MENTAL ILLNESSES AND TREATMENTS

BUILDING MENTAL HEALTH CAPACITY IN HAITI THROUGH COLLABORATIVE PARTNERSHIPS

MENTAL ILLNESSES AND TREATMENTS

Additional books in this series can be found on Nova's website
under the Series tab.

Additional e-books in this series can be found on Nova's website
under e-books tab.

MENTAL ILLNESSES AND TREATMENTS

BUILDING MENTAL HEALTH CAPACITY IN HAITI THROUGH COLLABORATIVE PARTNERSHIPS

GUERDA NICOLAS
GEMIMA ST. LOUIS
AND
CASTAGNA LACET

NOVINKA

New York

NOTICE TO THE READER

Additional color graphics may be available in the e-book version of this book.

Library of Congress Cataloging-in-Publication Data

ISBN: 978-1-63485-169-5

Library of Congress Control Number: 2016936932

Published by Nova Science Publishers, Inc. † New York

CONTENTS

PREFACE

As mental health providers of Haitian descent, we felt a calling to address such needs in our native home. However, we wanted to do so in a way that was respectful, culturally relevant, and useful. More importantly, we wanted to ensure that our efforts would not undermine, but would rather compliment, the work that our counterparts were implementing in the country. The material presented in this book is a result of our long-standing commitment to building mental health capacity and sustainability in Haiti through the development of a collaborative mental health training program over the past two decades. The focus of our work has been on ensuring the development and implementation of the program efficiently and effectively in different parts of the country. However, with the rise in the frequency of natural disasters occurring globally and the increase in the number of mental health professionals flying to different parts of the world to provide assistance during such times, it became more apparent that the experiences and lessons that we have learned from our work in Haiti might be beneficial to other mental health professionals looking to extend their work at the international level. The impetus for writing the book came after the first author (Dr. Guerda Nicolas) gave a keynote lecture at the Teachers' College Multicultural Roundtable during which she presented on the guiding principles of the mental health training program in Haiti. After the talk, many individuals approached her asking for more information about the program and the methods that were used. It was surprising to see that what appeared to have been common sense to us in conducting the program were novel ideas and approaches for others. We subsequently wrote an article about the approach in the Newsletter of the Office of International Affairs of the American Psychological Association that sparked more inquiries from different groups of professionals. The mental health training program have been integrated into the projects of Rebati Sante Mentale, an organization created by Haitians for Haitians focusing on building mental health capacity in Haiti and in the diaspora. Collectively, these experiences forced us to think about the need to publish a book that could be accessed by more individuals.

The book is written and intended for mental health professionals who are interesting in working at the international level. We hope that the information provided in the book will assist them in making informed decisions that are beneficial to the community of interest as well as for their own professional development. Although short-term work might be fulfilling for the implementer of a program, sustainable work creates a lasting legacy of the work to the benefit of the local community. We hope that the information provided in this book encourages the reader to pause before booking a flight to the next country in need of mental health services. Careful and thoughtful preparation will yield greater success for all stakeholders involved.

The writing of this book is a reflection of the sheer dedication of a group of trainers in Haiti and the U.S. who gave their time and talent on a monthly basis to ensure the successful implementation of the program. None of the individuals who have been involved with the project are employed through the project and all of them have full-time positions outside of the project. Thus, we are in awe of the unwavering dedication of the team of trainers in Ti Goave, Cap-Haitien, and Arcahaie who keep the program running year after year. THANK YOU for all that you do!

The writing of this book is also a testament to the many individuals who have dedicated their time to facilitate the training and to the countless number of teachers, nurses, doctors, and faith-based and community leaders who have participated in the training program. The publication of this book gives voice to your collective efforts and commitment to building a community consisting of individuals with "bon espri" (mental well-being). We are aware that the development of any community without a focus on building the psyche of its people can only lead to fruitless efforts that will not be sustainable over time. We hope that other communities and countries will benefit from the many lessons that we have learned from engaging in collaborative partnerships and doing this rewarding work in Haiti over the past 20 years.

Chapter 1

INTRODUCTION

Increasing disasters across the globe have led to increased interventions from international organizations to provide aid to the various countries that are in need of assistance (Lund et al., 2011). Such disasters are compounded by the high rate of poverty and mental health problems observed in these countries (Lund et al., 2011; Patel, 2007; Patel & Kleinman, 2003). Many low- and middle-income countries (LMICs) are not equipped with the resources to respond to this growing mental health challenge (Lund et al., 2011; Saraceno, Van Ommeren, Batniji, Cohen, Gureje, & Mahoney, 2007; Wang, Berglund, & Olfson, 2004. As a short-term solution, many mental health workers from the international community often travel to these countries to provide assistance and fill this gap; however, these initiatives alone cannot lead to sustainable programming in the regions served. The increasing focus on mental health across the globe calls for guidance on how mental disorders manifest across different cultures and best practice models for addressing these issues from a cultural context.

Additionally, in countries with limited resources and increased susceptibility to natural disasters, the call is even more urgent. In addition to poverty and limited resources, LMICs are most vulnerable to disasters, which make the need for culturally sensitive and sustainable mental health programs even greater. A recent example is the devastating Typhoon Haiyan, which occurred in the Philippines, a country classified as low-middle income (WHO, 2015).

While mental health providers may be rushed to provide assistance, or propelled to respond to mental health needs of LMICs, we must first stop and ensure that what we will be doing is necessary and grounded within the culture of the country. This monograph provides a framework for how to address mental health issues internationally in collaboration with local partners to create sustainable programs. Specifically, the monograph provides didactic and practical examples using a mental health-training program that has been implemented in Haiti for the past 20 years. Successes and challenges, as well as lessons learned and recommendations for other practitioners and researchers are provided.

Role of NGOs in Addressing Mental Health Needs in Low- and Middle-Income Countries

The preponderance of international Non-Governmental Organizations (NGOs) serves as an indication of the international community's desire to respond to the mental health needs. In Guatemala, for example, there are 725 NGOs, of which 469 are category six (central sector organizations or CSOs) (Barr, Fafchamps, & Owens, 2005; Hansmann, 1980). In Haiti, which reportedly has the highest number of NGOs per capita, there are 549 NGOs, of which 379 are CSOs, compared to just 190 (44 CSOs) in Trinidad and 219 (74 CSOs) in Jamaica (Schuller, 2012). While the needs are obvious and LMICs can benefit significantly from assistance from the international community, studies suggest that at times NGOs may do more harm than good in the locality (Garonne, 2011; Saraceno, van Ommeren, Batniji, Cohen, Gureje, Mahoney, Sridhar, & Underhill, 2007; Schuller, 2012). Garonne (2011) warns that harm may occur unintentionally through decreasing the local economy (purchasing materials out of the country instead in the country), providing service delivery that harms the health and wellbeing of the local people (providing services that are not culturally relevant or appropriate), and by reinforcing conflict (working with some stakeholders and not others can fuse existing conflicts between some organizations or the people and the government). NGOs may also weaken established local infrastructure, such as local NGOs, by removing able workers from more effective local positions due to increased opportunities. Garonne (2011) further cautions that insufficient pre-departure research can lead to interventions by INGOs going awry. With respect to mental health, the issue of providing potentially harmful service can easily become a major problem. When persons are unfamiliar with the cultural context and impose culturally insensitive or irrelevant health care through the use of diagnostics, measures, and an overall approach that conveys lack of research, the risk of harm by those trained in mental health abroad increases. These concerns notwithstanding, it is irresponsible to deny the needs of low- and middle-income countries. NGOs can offer much needed support in such resource-starved contexts.

Researchers, practitioners, and policy makers in Latin America and the Caribbean emphasize the need for historical and sociocultural frameworks to improve the mental health realities of the region's peoples (e.g., Beaubrun, 1992; Pan American Health Organization [PAHO], 2009; Ward & Hickling, 2004); however, they readily acknowledge the paucity of published materials that document the nature and extent of mental health disorders in the region (Hickling, 2005; PAHO, 2008). In its 2010 mental health strategic plan, PAHO highlighted gaps in basic mental health information, mental health resources, and treatment (PAHO, 2009). These limitations increase the burden of mental illness (PAHO, 2008) and compromise the overall health and well-being of the region's citizens, as mental health resources are also vital in addressing a myriad of psychosocial challenges, including traumatic experiences and natural disasters (PAHO, 2009). Several countries around the world are working to close the treatment gap using a range of best practices.

The World Health Organization recently published an overview of best practices in various countries around the world with a focus on integrated mental health, which has been shown to yield positive outcomes (WHO, 2011). Countries reviewed include Argentina, Australia, Belize, Brazil, India, Iran, Saudi Arabia, South Africa, Uganda, and the United Kingdom. Of the countries reviewed, only Belize, India, and Uganda fall into the World Bank's low- and middle-income categories. Since there is overlap in the types of challenges that many LMICs face, a review of models employed by low- and middle-income countries might provide further insight into strategies for health care related NGOs and professionals in approaching development work in LMICs.

Best Practice Mental Health Programs in Low- and Middle-Income Countries

As the previous section denotes, the mental health needs in low-income countries such as Haiti are vast and are often unique to a country's particular cultural nuances. Yet, while the needs in such countries may be heavily influenced by their cultural context, much insight can be gained from exploring other existing international interventions and the unique cultural and socio-political contexts in which they are implemented. In this vein, the following section provides an overview of some successful models reported in the WHO report (2011) used to implement mental health programming internationally.

Best Practice: Uganda

In Uganda, a low-income country where it is estimated that only half of the population has ready access to health care, health authorities implemented a model of integration in the district of Sembabule (World Health Organization and World Organization of Family Doctors, 2008). In this model, primary care workers identified, assessed, and treated common mental disorders and stable chronic disorders, referring patients as necessary. Uganda's primary health care system consists of several levels of care, each of which is staffed by various health care professionals. At the lowest level, staff may include nurses or midwives with assistants who have no formal training, while the highest level includes general doctors, psychiatric nurses, and more. The model was infused through all levels of health care and subsequently provided for ongoing mentoring and training of primary health care workers through specialist outreach services. Training also occurred on multiple levels. Health workers were trained in basic epidemiological knowledge and also received ongoing training around broader issues like managing difficult cases and building confidence for nurses. One unique and culturally specific characteristic of the approach was the incorporation of village health teams, trained volunteers from the village who help identify, refer, and monitor people with mental disorders. Village health teams played the crucial role of identifying and referring persons in the community who would otherwise be left untreated and also monitored those persons who were receiving treatment.

Some additional key characteristics of Uganda's model include the formation of a consumer association for the purpose of patient support and advocacy, and inclusion of mental health in the information system to increase awareness of mental disorders and their importance. Overall, the integration of mental health into general health care resulted in services that are more accessible, affordable, available, and acceptable through treating patients in their own communities. Important to note is that Ugandan authorities provided strong political support for mental health. Prior to implementation, political leaders, district health managers, and general health workers were all trained to address various issues including stigmatic attitudes and information about the new policy, with the goal of getting buy-in from stakeholders. This was conducted largely to address issues of stigma, which had historically limited treatment seeking for persons with common mental disorders. After implementation, however, health care workers recognized their responsibility in treating patients with mental illness. Attitudes of political leaders also shifted to an understanding of the importance of mental health. Some challenges to the Uganda's initiative included high patient demand, initial resistance to training due to strained human resources, stigmatic attitudes that persisted among health workers, and access to medicines that were not available on a regular basis in sufficient supply.

While models such as the one described from Uganda give insight into best practice principles that can be translated to other countries, it is important to note that diversity amongst and within countries call for a diversity of models. With the exception of Belize, Caribbean models of integration are scarce and due to limited resources, low- and middle-income countries are also not well represented in the literature.

Best Practice: Belize

In the low-income country of Belize, a two-stage approach was taken to increase providers' skills through a nation-wide district-based integration of mental health care. Belize's primary care infrastructure is made up of three polyclinics, 37 health centers, 43 public rural health stations, and eight government hospitals, including the country's sole national mental health hospital (World Health Organization & World Organization of Family Doctors, 2008). The health centers are responsible for providing general health education, immunization services, and ambulatory services, as well as providing outreach services in the form of mobile clinics and community nursing aides. Seven of the eight district hospitals are staffed by two psychiatric nurses who are responsible for providing mental health services, typically with one nurse stationed at the hospital while the second focuses on more community outreach services. The mental health services offered are community geared and provide preventive mental health care, crisis management, outpatient services, and other outreach services. In Belize, psychiatry is slowly gaining acceptance, with the position of the psychiatric nurse expanding to provide counseling to patients who are experiencing mental distress.

In 1992, the Ministry of Health began a two-stage approach to mental health care integration. Prior to the new paradigm of mental health, Belize relied on psychiatrists from other countries to work for two-year contracts in order to fill the country's professional gap. Recognizing that it was necessary to develop skills at the district level prior to implementing fully integrated primary care services, the Ministry selected a cohort of 16 psychiatric nurse practitioners who would help train the general practitioners. The original cohort represented all the district hospitals at the launch of their integration plan. At the end of the 10-month training program, the nurses returned to their hospitals under the ongoing supervision of psychiatrists in order to establish a permanent presence of mental health services in the hospitals. This was accomplished through more consistent and organized mental health care, as well as through the provision of services that were more strongly community-oriented. The psychiatric nurse practitioners conducted outpatient clinics, as well mental health education in schools and communities. By means of an ongoing partnership with PAHO, Belize has trained nearly 75% of their psychiatric nurse practitioners in the 10-month program. Nurse practitioners have also been given additional prescription rights. In the second phase of Belize's mental health integration, the program will focus on strengthening psychiatric nurse practitioners' direct interactions with primary care providers, in order to train them to manage mental health issues and conditions within their general practices.

Some key characteristics of Belize's model are the district health teams that consist of a psychiatric nurse, general practitioners, public health nurses, and community nurse aides. On such teams, the psychiatric nurse is referred to for training in mental health issues and provides other team members with on-going training. These teams helped to decentralize Belize's mental healthcare system by increasing outpatient services and creating community-based mental health prevention and promotion programs. Although this approach has not resulted in a fully integrated mental health service system, it has increased treatment coverage of individuals with mental disorders through outpatient services. Through this approach it was revealed that although some patients require referral to psychiatrists, a nurse trained in psychiatry can successfully address most mental health issues.

Best Practice: Ghana

The country of Ghana's approach to integrating health care was first addressed at the policy level. In collaboration with the WHO, In March 2012 Ghana developed and passed a Mental Health Bill to replace their 1972 mental health law (Doku, Wusu-Taky, & Awakame, 2012). While the old law placed a strong emphasis on institutional care and often went against international human rights standards, the new law will protect the rights of people with mental disorders and promote community based mental health care. The Mental Health Bill was developed through training workshops, consultations with key stakeholders, and critical analyses using WHO materials and tools. Overall, the health system is decentralized from the national, regional, and district levels (WHO, 2007a). Among its aims, the new law sought to improve access to inpatient and outpatient mental health care, and promote voluntary versus arbitrary involuntary mental health treatment.

Prior to passing the new bill, mental health services in Ghana took place primarily in the country's three public psychiatric hospitals, four private psychiatric hospitals, and 10 regional hospitals. Since the passing of the 2012 Bill, community psychiatric nurses (CPNs) have received further training in community care and are based in the main district. Of Ghana's 138 districts, 69 are served by at least one CPN, whose roles are to provide and identify cases of mental issues and to follow-up on the patient's use of psychotropic medications. In three of its regions, Ghana makes use of psychiatric diplomats, general doctors with 18 months training in psychiatry. Aside from the public services described above, Ghana also utilizes private sector facilities and NGOs in the delivery of mental health services.

As demonstrated by the Uganda, Belize, and Ghana systems of care outlined above, models for integrating mental health care into primary health care should look different from place to place. The design and implementation of these models should be based on the various cultural needs and challenges specific to the mental health (and other) needs of a country, such as the structure of the healthcare system, the reach and impact of stigma surrounding mental health, and more. The key principles that underlie these best practices should be noted and applied to international mental health programming when appropriate. In their report on integrating mental health into primary care, the World Health Organization and the World Organization of Family Doctors (2008) draw from a number of best practices to outline several principles to guide the work (see Table 1). The principles outlined by the WHO focus on strategies for integrating mental health into primary care. In a similar manner, this monograph aims to add to the body of literature on best practice models for conducting mental health programming in low- and middle-income countries. Specifically, we will focus on programming that fosters mental health capacity building using examples from the design and implementation of Haiti-based projects.

BRIEF OVERVIEW OF THE MENTAL HEALTH TRAINING PROGRAM IN HAITI

The purpose of the mental health-training program is to provide the necessary resources and support to:

1. Increase capacity and sustainability of mental health in Haiti by training health professionals and community psychosocial counselors in psychosocial programming and implementation.
2. Train health professionals and community leaders to recognize symptoms of psychological distress in individuals.
3. Train health professionals and community leaders to become trainers on how to conduct information sessions with other groups in their respective communities.
4. Increase community awareness about mental health issues and ways of seeking services for these issues through the "train-the-trainer" model.

The specific aims of the mental health training component are to: a) train and provide ongoing support for health care providers, teachers, and community health workers in Haiti to identify, screen for, and offer support for mental health needs of patients; b) prepare a selected group of trainees to become trainers in identifying, screening for, and offering mental health support; and c) prepare selected health providers to provide more intensive services to patients. Training is conducted in a five-day course. The program has been culturally adapted for use with Haitians, linguistically translated, and employed successfully in Haiti following a natural disaster. The developer of the cultural adaptation is Dr. Guerda Nicolas, a Haitian-American psychologist. Dr. Nicolas directs the mental health component for the project and provides training and supervision. Below we provide an overview of the mental health-training program in Haiti that will be illustrated throughout the book.

The program has been applied both in crisis and general care, and was adapted for use in response to hurricanes (Nicolas, DeSilva, Houlahan, & Beltrame, 2009) and the 2010 earthquake in Haiti. The training manual presents basic concepts in understanding disaster-related behaviors to explain phases of such behaviors and outline post-disaster intervention strategies for mental health problems. The manual is divided into the following sections: (1) conceptualizations of basic concepts in understanding disaster behavior, focusing on stress resulting from the crisis, social supports at the time of the crisis, and coping skills of the individual victim; (2) phases of disaster-related behaviors, illustrated by a table listing typical reactions to stress for preschoolers, latency age children, preadolescents and adolescents, adults, and senior citizens; and (3) post-disaster intervention strategies for mental health problems in the acute phase, including mental illness, drug abuse, alcohol problems, and disaster worker stress. This training is supplemented by Tucker's (2007) patient-centered culturally sensitive health care model (PCCSHCM) that involves the following components: (a) training health care providers and office staff to engage in behaviors and display attitudes that make patients feel comfortable with, trusting of, and respected by the health care professionals involved in their treatment; (b) modifying the physical environment of the health care facility so that patients feel welcome there; and (c) training patients in behaviors and skills that increase the likelihood that they will be treated in a culturally sensitive manner by the health care professionals involved in their treatment.

This program has been implemented in Haiti and shown to be effective in increasing participants' recognition of symptoms of mental health issues, and improving individuals' perception of mental disorders, efficiency, and self-efficacy. We have conducted this training in various sectors of the country with different professional groups (e.g., physicians, nurses, religious leaders, teachers, and community leaders).

The mental health-training program has a built-in evaluation component. Personnel are evaluated on their knowledge base and their awareness of psychological issues at the beginning of the training, midway through program, at program completion, and at follow-up booster sessions using a quantifiable questionnaire. A measure of psychological distress developed for the program is also administered to the participants (Nicolas, Artnz, Hirsch, & Schmiedigen, 2009).

Training of Trainers

Part of the training protocol involves selecting a set of individuals who will receive additional training to serve as health educators to conduct the training program, thus ensuring an enduring capacity for addressing mental health in the region. The program has a capacity-building component that is both systemic and regional in nature, enabling the sustainability of the program. The specific details regarding the sustainability of the program can be found in chapter 5 of the monograph.

Evaluation of the Project

Processes for evaluating the impact of the project and for detailing lessons learned in implementing this training program are a high priority. Some quantitative elements that we aim to use in the program evaluation include:

1. The administration of pre/posttest questionnaires to collect data on knowledge and psychological distress for the mental health component
2. Assessment of competencies gained through training
3. Measures of participants' satisfaction with training and services

In addition to the quantitative assessment, we conducted interviews and focus groups to gauge the impact of and satisfaction with the project. Of particular interest are issues of cultural competence and satisfaction of the personnel with respect to their participation in the project. Dr. Nicolas, a researcher with over 20 years of experiences, directs the planning and implementation of the program evaluation. The evaluation plan is designed in close consultation with other key personnel and after first-hand observation of the facilities and resources. See chapter 6 for more details about the evaluation approach and methods use for the training program.

Overview of the Monograph

This monograph is a guidebook focusing on how to implement mental health training programs internationally. The book is structured in a way that utilizes Haiti as an example of what scholars who are interested in global mental health can do to effectively implement a training program internationally. As such, the monograph includes didactic information as well as detailed practical examples with illustrations of the experience in implementing our mental health training program in Haiti for the past 20 years. The book opens with the guiding principles that we have used as a framework for our work: (1) In-Country Partnership; (2) Enhancing Cultural Knowledge; (3) Building a Culturally Competent team; (4) Building Culturally Relevant Curriculum; and (5) Building Capacity. The subsequent chapters show the reader how to use the framework and approaches for adaptation to any subject and country.

This monograph is intended for practitioners, academics, researchers, human service providers, program administrators, public health advocates, policymakers, community leaders, undergraduate and graduate students, non-profit and grassroots organizations, and state and international agencies with an interest in developing, implementing, and evaluating culturally-appropriate mental health training programs for use in international settings. Given the increasing number of individuals immigrating to the United States and the increasing diversity of the demographic composition of the country, the information presented in this monograph can also be useful within the United States to individuals who are interested in learning about ways to make mental health programs more culturally appropriate to ethnically diverse clients. We recognize that there are many great examples of how to effectively implement a mental health training program internationally, thus, this book is not an attempt to represent all of these perspectives, or to indicate that ours is unique. We simply provide an example of one type of mental health training program that has been working effectively and sustainably over the past 20 years in Haiti, and hope that it will be useful to many colleagues who seek to engage in similar work.

REFERENCES

Barr, A., Marcel, F., & Trudy, O (2005). "The Governance of Non-Governmental Organizations in Uganda." *World Development*, 33(4), 657-79, April.

Doku, V.C.K., Wusu-Taky, A., & Awakame, J. (2012). Implementing the mental health act in Ghana: Any challenges ahead? *Ghana Medical Journal*, *46*, 241-250.

Hansmann, Henry. 1980. "The Role of Nonprofit Enterprise." *The Yale Law Journal*, 89, no. 5 (April).

Lund, C., DeSilva, M., Plagerson, S., Cooper, S., et al. (2011). Poverty and mental disorders: Breaking the cycle in low-income and middle-income countries. *Lancet*, 378 (9801), 1502-1514.

Patel, V., & Kleinman, A. (2003). Poverty and common mental disorders in developing countries. Bulletin of the World Health Organization, 81(8), 609-615.

Patel, V., Kirkwood, B. R., Pednekar, S., Weiss, H. & Mabey, D. 2006. Risk factors for common mental disorders in women. Population-based longitudinal study. *British Journal of Psychiatry*, *189*, 547-55.

Roberts, M., Mogan, C., & Asare, J.B. (2014) An overview of Ghana's mental health system: results from an assessment using the world health organization's assessment instrument for mental health systems (WHO-AIMS). *International Journal of Mental Health System*, 8 (16). doi:10.1186/1752-4458-8-16.

Saraceno B, van Ommeren M, Batniji R, Cohen A, Gureje O, Mahoney J, Sridhar D, Underhill C (2007) Barriers to improvement of mental health services in low-income and middle-income countries. *Lancet*, 370, 1164–1174. doi:10.1016/S0140-6736(07)61263-X.

Saraceno B., Van Ommeren M., Batniji R., Cohen A., Gureje O., Mahoney J. (2007). Barriers to improvement of mental health services in low-income and middle-income countries. *Lancet*, *370*, 1164–1174.

Schuller, M. (2012). Killing with Kindness: Haiti, International Aid, and NGOs. New Brunswick, NJ: Rutgers University Press, xvi+233 pp.

Sharan, P; Gallo, C; Gureje, O; Lamberte, E; Mari, JJ; Mazzotti, G; Patel, V; Swartz, L; Olifson, S; Levav, I; de Francisco, A; Saxena, S; World Hlth Org-Global Forum Hlth, R (2009) Mental health research priorities in low- and middle-income countries of Africa, Asia, Latin America and the Caribbean. *The British Journal of Psychiatry*, *195* (4). pp. 354-363. ISSN 0007-1250 Downloaded from: http://researchonline.lshtm.ac.uk/4563/

Sipsma H, Ofori-Atta A, Canavan M, Osei-Akoto I, Udry C, Bradley EH (2013) Poor mental health in Ghana: who is at risk? *BMC Public Health*, 13 (288). doi:10.1186/1471-2458-13-288.

Wang, P.S., Berglund, P.A., Olfson, M., et al. (2004). Delays in initial treatment contact after first onset of a mental disorder. *Health Service Research*, *39*, 393–415.

World Health Organization (2010a). Mental health and development: targeting people with mental health conditions as a vulnerable group, Geneva, WHO Press.

World Health Organization (2010b). WHO: mhGAP intervention guide for mental, neurological and substance use disorders in non-specialized health settings. http://www.who.int/mental_health/publications/mhGAP_intervention_guide/en/. Accessed 6 Jun 2015.

World Health Organization (2011) WHO-AIMS report on mental health system in Ghana. http://www.who.int/mental_health/who_aims_country_reports/ghana_who_aims_report.pdf?ua=1. Accessed January 2015.

Chapter 2

THE MENTAL HEALTH TRAINING PROGRAM COMPONENTS

"Our definitions and treatments have become the international standards. Although this has often been done with the best of intentions, we've failed to foresee the full impact of these efforts. It turns out that how a people in a culture think about mental illnesses – how they categorize and prioritize the symptoms, attempt to heal them, and set expectations for their course and outcome – influences the diseases themselves. In teaching the rest of the world to think like us, we have been, for better and worse, homogenizing the way the world goes mad."

Ethan Watters,
Crazy Like Us: The Globalization of the American Psyche

In 1978, the World Health Organization requested that governments in the Caribbean study and implement both traditional and Western medicine strategies as part of a national primary health care initiative. This call was repeated by the Pan American Health Organization (PAHO, 2007) and supported by international organizations invested in increasing access to quality health care throughout the Latin American and Caribbean region (LAC). Yet, a more comprehensive health care initiative is needed to address the unmet health needs of the Haitian people. Sociopolitical and socioeconomic factors, as well as cultural beliefs and customs, greatly influence the health of Haitian individuals. For example, certain mental health disorders or culturally-bound syndromes (e.g., *move san* and *sezisman*) are believed to be caused by fright or exposure of childbearing women to negative emotions (Miller, 2000; Nicolas, DeSilva, Grey, & Gonzalez-Eastep, 2006). Women who suffer from *move san* ("bad blood") or *sezisman* (fright or shock) are likely to experience weakness and skin eruptions, spoiled breast milk, headaches and depression, miscarriage or premature delivery, state of paralysis, and even death (Miller, 2000). Thus, any mental health training program must take into these cultural elements and ensure an indigenous understanding of the symptoms and disorders. In this chapter, we provide a detailed description of the mental health training program that has been implemented in Haiti for the past 20 years.

Overview of the Mental Health Training Program

The main objectives of the mental health training component are to:

a) Train and provide ongoing support for health care providers, teachers, and community health workers in Haiti to identify, screen for, and offer support for mental health needs of patients;
b) Prepare a selected group of trainees to become trainers in identifying, screening for, and offering mental health support; and
c) Prepare selected health providers to provide more intensive services to patients.

The program was designed for use with Haitians throughout the different regions of the country. It has been culturally adapted, linguistically translated, and employed successfully with community leaders, health care professionals, and teachers. The training program, which was culturally tailored for Haiti and developed by a Haitian psychologist, is intended to increase participants' knowledge of the common mental health symptoms experienced after a disaster or a traumatic experience; the manifestations of these symptoms for individuals across different ages, genders and cultures in Haiti; and culturally-tailored strategies to implementation with individuals who have experienced a traumatic life event. The implementation of this program was intended to enable professionals (e.g., health care providers and teachers) and community leaders to identify possible mental health symptoms in individuals so that they can offer support and knowledge, and facilitate access to care.

The developer of the training program, Dr. Guerda Nicolas, is a Haitian-American psychologist who directs the mental health component of the project and provides training and supervision to trainers. She leads a team composed of Haitian-American mental health professionals, including psychiatrists, psychologists, social workers, nurses, and mental health counselors, all of whom are experienced in disaster response and in providing mental health services to culturally-diverse populations.

THEORETICAL APPROACH: A FOCUS ON WELLNESS AND CULTURAL COMPETENCY

The well-being perspective and the WHO definition of mental health guide the Mental Health Training Program "mental health is a state of *well-being* in which every individual realizes his or her own potential, can cope with the normal stresses of life, can work productively and fruitfully, and is able to make a contribution to her or his community" (WHO, 1978). This definition is further supported by the evidence based framework and holistic principles outlined by Dr. Isaac Prilleltensky. Prilleltensky (1994a) has detailed how parents, schools, communities and social policy makers can enact these values for the promotion of child and family wellness. BET I CAN is an acronym for seven factors that work together to understand and improve well-being:

- Behavior
- Emotions
- Thoughts
- Interactions
- Context
- Awareness
- Next Steps

According to Muñoz, Mrazek, and Haggerty (1996), "Mental health promotion entails more than seeking freedom from disorders or ailments. It represents attempts to seek a sense of coherence, health, wellness, zest, resilience, self-efficacy, empowerment, energy, flexibility, order, balance, harmony, and integrity" (p. 1121). In *Mental health for Canadians: Striking a balance*, psychological wellness is defined as follows:

> Mental health is the capacity of the individual, the group and the environment to interact with one another in ways that promote subjective well-being, the optimal development and use of mental abilities (cognitive, affective, and

> relational), the achievement of individual and collective goals consistent with justice and the attainment and preservation of conditions of fundamental equality. (Epp, 1988, p. 7)

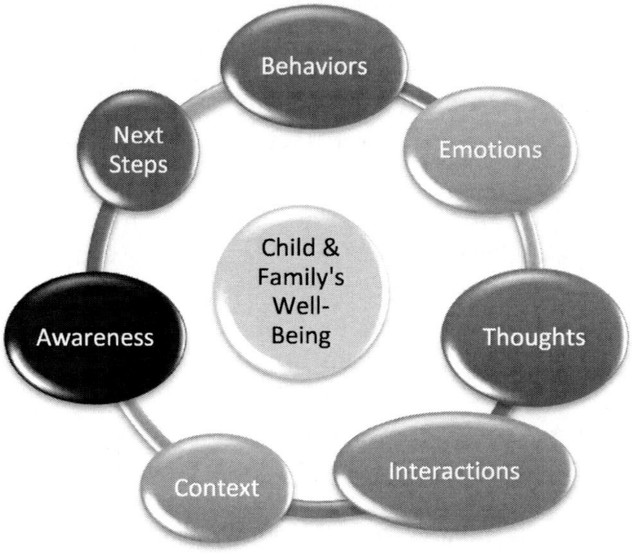

Figure 1

Wellness is not the same as the absence of disease. Rather, it is defined by the presence of positive markers characterize by a combination of personality, family, community and social elements. Collectively, these elements can serve as a buffer against the development of mental health problems. Thus, focusing on wellness centers on prevention rather risk-driven interventions (Cowen, 1996).

At the other end of the health continuum we find risks and deficits. Historically, most efforts and investments in the physical and mental health fields have been directed toward the reduction of risks and the correction of deficits. When the primary mandate of health professionals is to fix problems, not to avert them, little attention is paid to wellness promotion, even though it is a more humane and cost efficient method of securing health and safety (Albee, 1996; Cowen, 1996).

Risk reduction is a very legitimate endeavor, but it has to be balanced with strategies to promote well-being. In promoting life satisfaction, we build a buffer zone against stressful events and transitions. Hence, we diminish the chances of negative chain reactions when faced with adverse circumstances.

Wellness enhancement is an ongoing task; it is part of a deliberate plan to achieve optimum health and satisfaction through the actualization of personal and social values. This entails the promotion of values such as caring, the protection of health, education and personal development, self-determination, and social justice. Prilleltensky (1994) has detailed how parents, schools, communities, and social policymakers can enact these values for the promotion of child and family wellness.

In addition to the focus on promoting health and wellness, the Haitian Mental Health Training Program is supplemented by the patient-centered culturally sensitive health care model (PCCSHCM). Introduced by Tucker and colleagues (2007), the PCCSHCM involves (a) training health care providers to engage in the behaviors and display the attitudes that make patients feel comfortable with, trusting of, and respected by the health care professionals involved in their treatment; (b) modifying the physical environment of the health care facility so that patients feel welcome there; and (c) training patients in behaviors and skills that increase the likelihood that they will be treated in a culturally sensitive manner by the health care professionals involved in their treatment. This program has been implemented in Haiti over the past two decades and shown to be effective in increasing participants' recognition of symptoms of mental health issues and improving individuals' perception of mental disorders and self-efficacy.

THE TRAINING PROGRAM

In this section, we provide an overview of the focus of the program. The purpose of the mental health training program is to provide the necessary resources and support to help health care providers, teachers, school directors, and community health workers. Thus, the training program aims to:

1. Increase capacity and sustainability of mental health services in Haiti by training health care professionals, teachers, and community psychosocial counselors in psychosocial programming and implementation
2. Train health professionals, teachers, and community leaders to recognize symptoms of psychological distress in individuals
3. Train health professionals, teachers, and community leaders to become trainers on how to conduct information sessions with other groups in their respective communities

4. Increase community awareness about mental health concerns and ways of seeking services for these issues through a "train-the-trainer" model.

The program has been applied in Haiti both in crisis and general care, and has been adapted for use in response to hurricanes (Nicolas, DeSilva, Houlahan, & Beltrame, 2009) and the January 2010 earthquake. The training manual presents basic concepts in understanding disaster-related behaviors to explain phases of such behaviors and outlines post-disaster intervention strategies for mental health problems. The manual includes discussions on the following: (1) conceptualizations of basic concepts in understanding disaster behavior, focusing on stress resulting from the crisis, social supports at the time of the crisis, and coping skills of the individual victim; (2) phases of disaster-related behaviors, illustrated by a table listing typical reactions to stress for preschoolers, latency age children, preadolescents and adolescents, adults, and senior citizens; and (3) post-disaster intervention strategies for mental health problems in the acute phase, including mental illness, drug abuse, alcohol problems, and disaster worker stress.

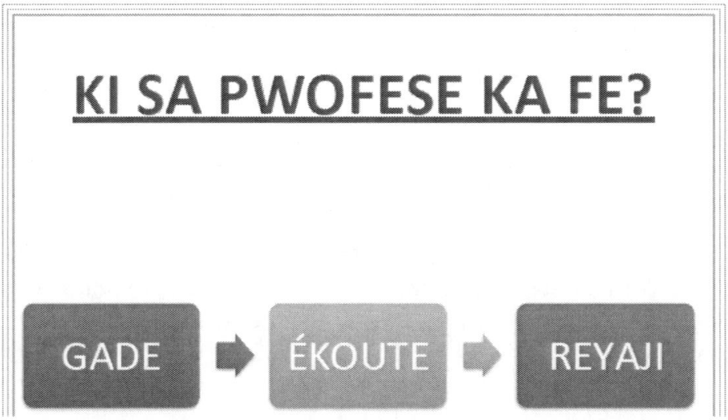

Figure 2. The Model of the Program.

The program is built around the concept of *Observe, Listen, and React* as illustrated in Figure 2. We aim at assisting the participants to become good observers of the people in their lives and to pay attention to any changes that they are seeing in behavior. It is the change in behavior that may warrant their attention. Second, we teach them the importance of listening. Upon observing changes in behavior, having a conversation with the individual where the focus is on listening to individual and not advice given is important. Lastly, we provide some tips of ways to react depending on the types of issues that the person is dealing. Ultimately, we want them to be able to intervene within their role and not taking on the role of a mental health provider.

Components of the Mental Health Training Program

The conceptual framework that guides the training program is described in chapter two of this monograph. In this section, we focus on the curriculum, the content of the training program, and the "train-the-trainer" model. The curriculum that is used for the program was created by members of the CRECER (*Challenging Racism and Empowering Communities through Ethnocultural Research*) team at the University of Miami's School of Education and Human Development, under the direction of Dr. Guerda Nicolas. The training manual can be used in training medical personnel, teachers, and community workers on the mental health issues pertaining to the Haitian community. The material provided in the manual is not an exhaustive list of information but a starting point for many who work with Haitians or who are planning to engage in capacity-building initiatives in Haiti.

The Curriculum

The curriculum, which has been translated into Haitian Kreyol, French, and English, serves as the primary training tool. See Figure 2 for a look at the Table of contents for the book. The manual includes an introduction that provides a brief background of the program along with a description of the training goals and objectives. It is divided into the following five sections:

1. *Conceptualization of Health* — This section addresses some of the cultural concepts of health and illness in the Haitian community. Based on the seminal work published by Colin and Paperwalla (1996), it examines how the traditional view of health is often linked to the body being in a state of equilibrium between "hot" or "cold", and highlights that the root causes of both physical and mental ailments may have a natural or supernatural origin. This section also includes a

list and description of culturally-bound syndromes that are common in the Haitian culture, including *sezisman, gaz, chalè*, and *pèdisyon*.

2. *Family Structure and Relationships* — This section focuses on the Haitian family structure and provides an overview of the roles and relationships among elders, children, and other members of the family.
3. *Folk Medicine* — In this section, the focus is on the use of spiritual healers and home-based remedies as culturally-sanctioned approaches to symptom management and care.
4. *Mental Health Fact Sheets* — This section provides a more comprehensive description of mental health-related conditions that affect children, adolescents, and adults. The topics covered include depression, anxiety, trauma, and grief. For each topic that is addressed, there is a discussion on the warning signs, risk factors, common reactions (differentiated among children and adults), and coping mechanisms. Additionally, this section addresses key differences between mental health and mental illness; differences between normal development and mental health problems in children and adolescents; differences between symptoms, syndromes, and disorders; and culturally-bound mental illnesses.
5. *Practice Cases* — This section of the manual includes some case scenarios of hypothetical children, adolescents, and adults who experience a range of mental health conditions. The vignettes are used to assist program participants in applying some of the key concepts discussed during the course of the training.
6. *References and Resources* — The manual concludes with a list of references and resources.

It must be noted that, given the heterogeneity that exists in the Haitian culture (e.g., there are geographical and cultural differences throughout the region) and as part of the capacity-building program design, our Haiti-based partners were encouraged to tailor various aspects of the curriculum to make it more culturally appropriate for their respective communities. As a result, adjustments have been made to the curriculum, which created opportunities for cross-collaboration and for program participants to: 1) increase their interaction with the curriculum, 2) demonstrate and strengthen their leadership capacity, and 3) increase their level of engagement during the training sessions.

SA KI NAN LIV LA

2

Figure 3. The Table of Contents of the Training Manual.

Format of the Training Sessions

For the initial training that occurs in a particular region, the U.S.-based team will facilitate the training, in collaboration with the in-country program coordinator. In subsequent training sessions, the goal is to allow local trainers to take the leadership and run the group workshops with the support (rather than direction) of the U.S.-based team.

The training is conducted over the course of five (5) days from 8:00 a.m. to 4:00 p.m., using a group workshop format composed of 15-20 individuals. See Figure 3 for a sample agenda. The program uses an interactive approach, which allows the participants ample opportunities to connect with each other and the training materials. Program participants are typically recruited from diverse backgrounds and represent different regions of the country. For example, the training sessions that were conducted in Cap-Haitien included doctors, nurses, and other health care personnel. However, the group workshops that took place in Arcahaie were primarily focused on teachers from both public and private schools and school administrators from rural and urban areas.

The 5-day training session typically begins with welcoming remarks and an overview of the program provided by Dr. Nicolas, an in-country program coordinator, and public officials representing the region. Program participants then introduce themselves (e.g., where they come from, their background, what they hope to learn from the training, etc.). This is followed by a review of the logistics of the 5-day training session where participants are invited to ask and clarify any questions or concerns that they may have. Participants are asked to complete a pre-evaluation form to assess their knowledge and understanding of the topics that will be addressed during the training. The findings from the program evaluation are presented in another section of this monograph.

On the first day of the training session, small groups of 4-5 individuals are formed, representing a diverse range of experiences and backgrounds. This format allows individuals to become better acquainted with each other and create stronger group cohesion, and enables collaborative alliances and friendships to emerge during the training. As individuals gather in their respective groups, they participate in a "getting-to-know-you" activity where they choose a name for their group that reflects their collective identity. From that point forward, the group is identified by that name. Once assigned, individuals remain with their group until the end of the training session.

Programme Santé Mentale

Arcahaie Projet

Mai 20-24, 2013

Ordre du Jour

LUNDI

8:00am	Prise de Contact Comment remplir les formulaires pré-atelier, Pre-test
8:30am	Bienvenue Maire Wilson-Arcahaie Pierre Imbert, Barr Foundation
9:00	Introduction Ms. Mireille Fombrun Dr. Guerda Nicolas Les Co-Formateurs Les Participants 10:00 – 12:00pm Introduction A La Section Causes de la Maladie Mentale Que Peut Faires Des Enseignants? Estime de Soi et le Concept de Soi
12:00 – 1pm	Pause Dejeuner
2:00pm to 3:30pm	Les Advertissements, Facteurs de risque, et Symptômes Psychologiques chez les Adultes et les Enfants: L'Anxiété
3:30pm	Evaluation du jour

MARDI

8:00am	Recaputulation
8:30am – 10:30am	Visite guidée du musée
10:00am – 12:00pm	Histoire D'Haiti
12:00pm – 1pm	**Pause Déjeuner; Photo de groupe**
2:00pm to 3:30pm	Application de l'histoire de l'enseignement des différents groupes d'âge
3:30pm	Evaluation du jour

MERCREDI

8:00am	Recaputulation
8:30am – 10:00am	Les Advertissements, Facteurs de Risque, et Symptômes Psychologiques chez les Adultes et les Enfants: **Dépression**

10:00am	**Pause-Café**
10:45 am – 1pm	Les Advertissements, Facteurs de risque, et Symptômes Psychologiques chez les Adultes et les Enfants: **Traumastime**
1:00 – 2pm	**Pause Déjeuner**
2:00pm to 3:30pm	**Traumatisme** continue
3:30pm	Evaluation du jour

JEUDI

8:00am	Recaputulation
8:30am – 10:00am	Les Advertissements, Facteurs de risque, et Symptômes Psychologiques chez les Adultes et les Enfants: **Chagrin & Adaptation**
10:00am	**Pause-Café**
10:45 am – 1pm	Discussion des Cas
1:00 – 2pm	**Pause Déjeuner**
2:00pm to 3:30pm	Preparation des Presentations
3:30pm	Evaluation du jour

VENDREDI

8:00am	Examen des participants
9:00am – 1:00pm	Presentation Pratique Par les membres de L'equipe
1:00 – 2pm	**Pause Dėjeuner**
2:00pm to 3:30pm	Presentation finale
3:30pm	Evaluation de la session par les participants du jour

CLÔTURE

Figure 4. An Agenda Example from the Training Program

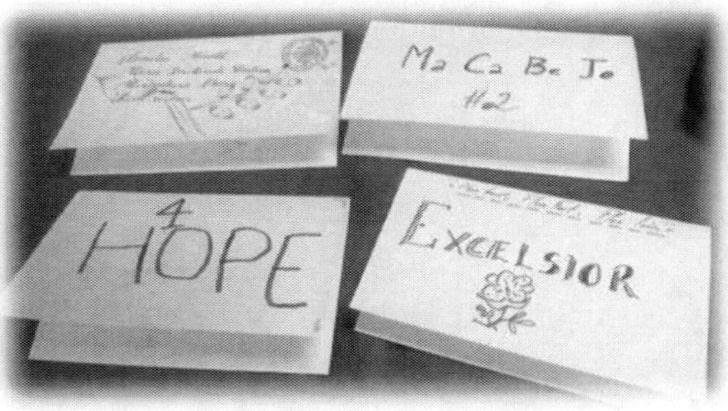

In order to allow program participants ample time to learn, discuss, process, and integrate the training materials, each day is devoted to a specific topic (e.g., depression, anxiety, trauma and grief). For instance, during the morning training session of a day devoted to anxiety, one team leader will facilitate a discussion on the types of commonly-occurring anxiety disorders among children and adolescents, followed by another leader addressing the cultural aspects of anxiety in terms of how it is manifested in the Haitian community. Participants then take a 1-hour lunch break where the conversations often continue within a collegial and interactive atmosphere. Lunch is always catered by a local restaurant that partners with the program. Participants and program leaders eat together and share stories about the local community and engage in informal discussions about life in their community. Following the lunch break, an afternoon training session occurs in a similar format as the morning group workshop. At the end of every day, participants are asked to complete an evaluation form to share their feedback on the activities of the day and provide input on what worked well and areas in need of improvement.

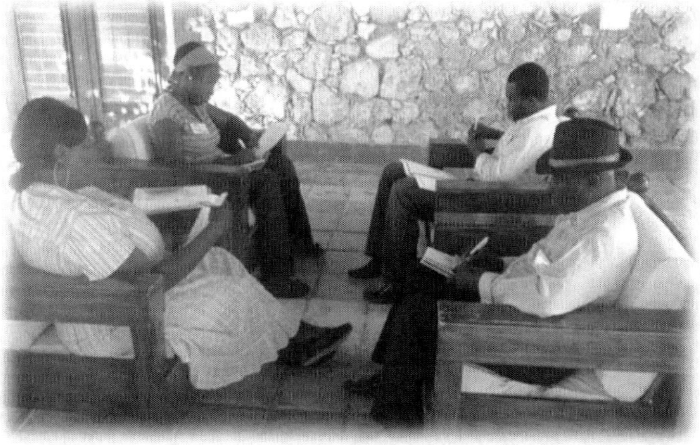

The following day, a new training session begins with welcoming remarks from trainers and a summary of the previous day's activities by one of the participants. A team leader then facilitates a group discussion on one of the training topics. As part of the participatory approach, participants are assigned specific sections (e.g., warning signs, risk factors, types of traumatic reactions, cultural factors, etc.) to review and discuss in their respective groups and then present to the larger audience. Vignettes are used to assist program participants in differentiating between symptoms of depression, anxiety, and trauma. Group members are encouraged to take charge of their assigned topics and actively engage in the discussion. The rest of the training session follows a similar format where all the main topics are covered and discussed.

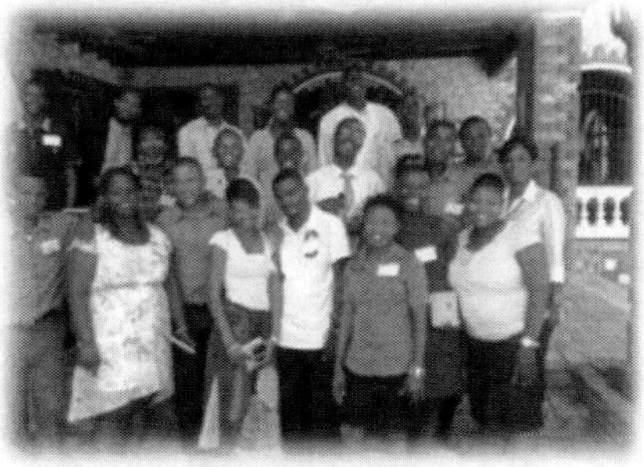
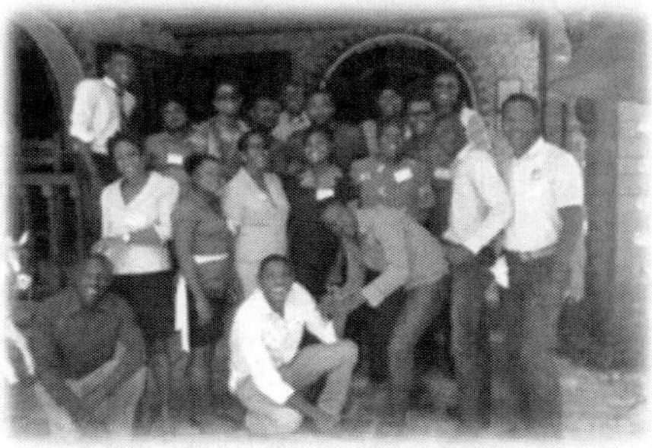
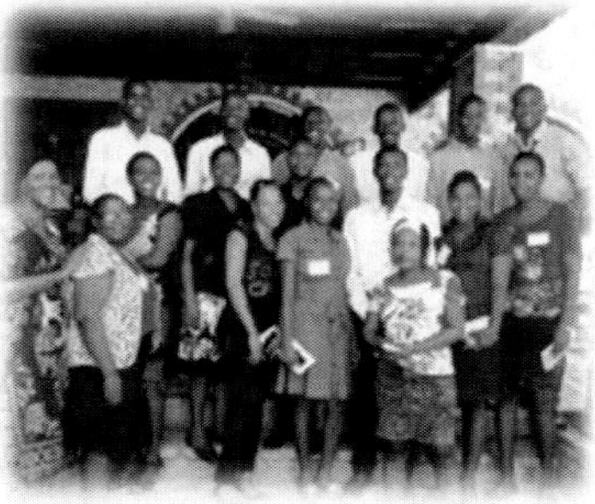
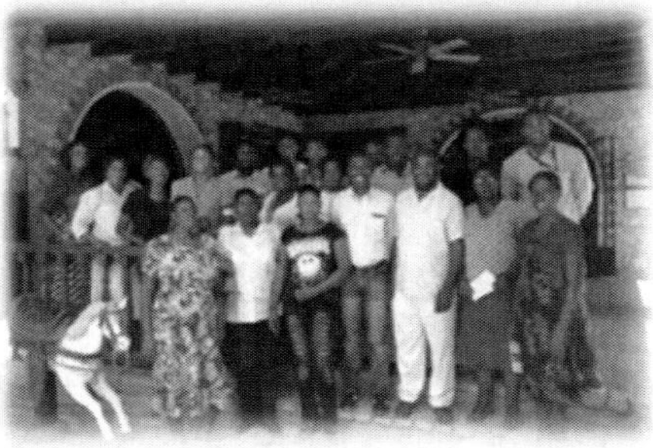

As noted earlier, the Haiti-based team was invited to make appropriate adjustments to the training program as well as its structure and format to ensure cultural sensitivity in the implementation of the model in various regions of the country. Below are some of the changes that the trainers recommended. Specifically, they adapted the program structure to include the following team-based roles and responsibilities:

1. The *Daily Recap Team* is responsible for reviewing the key aspects of the previous day's lesson each morning. Thus, trainers are given an opportunity to provide additional clarification on portions of the lesson that participants identify as being unclear.
2. The *Areas of Improvement Team* is responsible for identifying aspects of the previous day that could run more smoothly and effectively. This team provides the U.S.- and Haiti-based teams with insight into which programmatic areas need refining and can be addressed in future sessions. This feedback helps the participants feel that their concerns are not only being noted, but validated and addressed when appropriate.
3. The *Animation/Accolades Team* is responsible for the engagement of participants throughout the day. The team helps to foster a

supportive atmosphere by providing culturally relevant cheers and demonstrations of praise. These accolades help to provide a supportive learning environment for both trainers and participants.

4. The *Accountability Team* is responsible for creating a shared sense of accountability for the level of respect demonstrated throughout the sessions. The group encourages all participants to be responsible for the group's learning and the overall success of the training session.

These programmatic teams provide a culturally relevant way for participants to demonstrate and strengthen their leadership capacities. By supporting the development of these capacities, the trainers help to establish a strong sense of accountability, respect, and community within the training program.

On the last day of the group workshops, all participants give a group presentation based on a selected topic (i.e., depression, anxiety, trauma and grief). The day typically starts with one participant giving a full recap of all the activities that transpired during the week. Team leaders then provide some of the highlights based on the main topics discussed. The rest of the day is devoted to the group presentations. Some group members incorporate creative strategies into their presentations, including role-plays, skits, dance, and music. The group presentations are followed by an award ceremony where participants receive their certificates. All program participants then complete a post-assessment tool that measures their knowledge of the materials covered during the course of the group workshop.

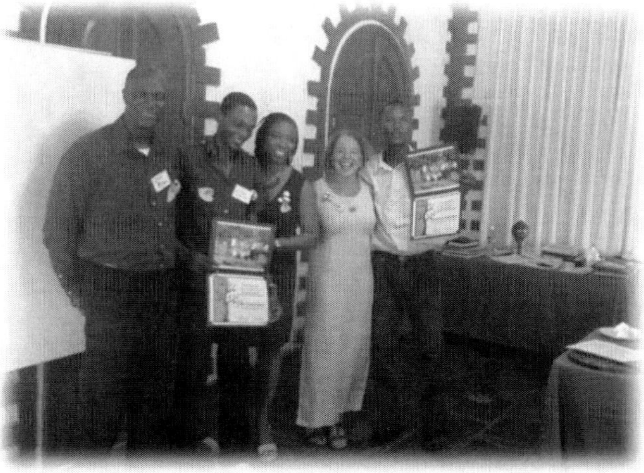

Adaptations

Of note are some elements that were incorporated into the training program conducted in Arcahaie, which enhanced the learning environment for program participants and reflected the cultural diversity of the context in which the training program occurred. First, as part of the training, all participants received a guided tour of the Ogier-Fombrun Museum (where the training took place) and an overview of the history of Haiti from pre-colonization to 1804. Prior to the tour, a group discussion was held on the links between the history of colonization, identity, and mental health and mental illness in Haiti. Second, at the start of each day, the group sang a spiritual song that brought them together and helped them to reflect on the activity of the day. Third, participants took turns leading program participants in a song/dance exercise during breaks to reduce fatigue and keep the focus on the task at hand. Lastly, participants provided great insight into cultural belief systems, values, traditions, and practices that were germane to understanding how mental illness was viewed and discussed in their respective communities.

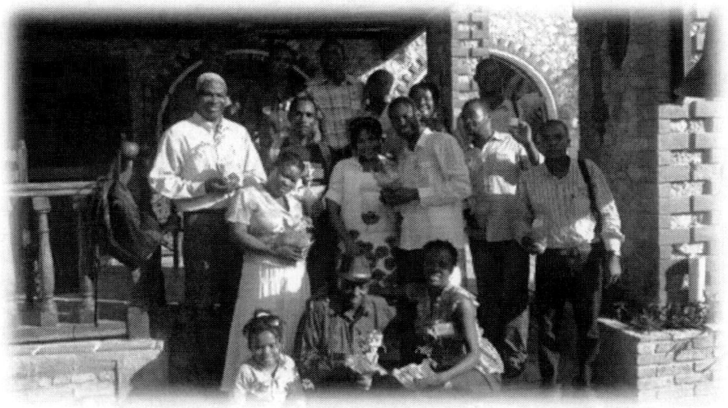

The "Train-the-Trainer" Model

Part of the training protocol involves selecting a set of individuals who will receive additional training to serve as health educators to conduct the training program, thus ensuring an enduring capacity for addressing mental health in the region. See Figure 5 for an overview of the trainer's manual used in the program.

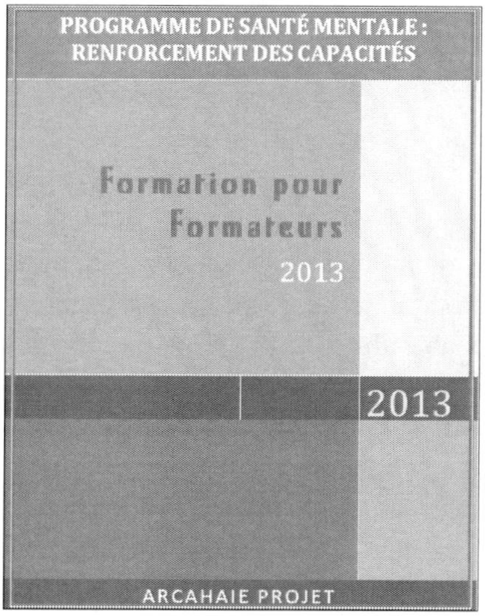

Figure 5. The Trainers Manual

Given that the primary focus of the training program is on capacity building, at the end of each training session a core group of 3-5 participants from various regions of the country are selected to receive additional training that will further prepare them to become trainers for future sessions. This mode l is guided by a participatory community empowerment approach, which aims to provide the necessary skills, knowledge, and training to educators and community leaders to enhance their ability to train others on the topics of mental health and mental illness. The program's capacity-building component is systemic in nature as well as regional, which enables the sustainability of the program.

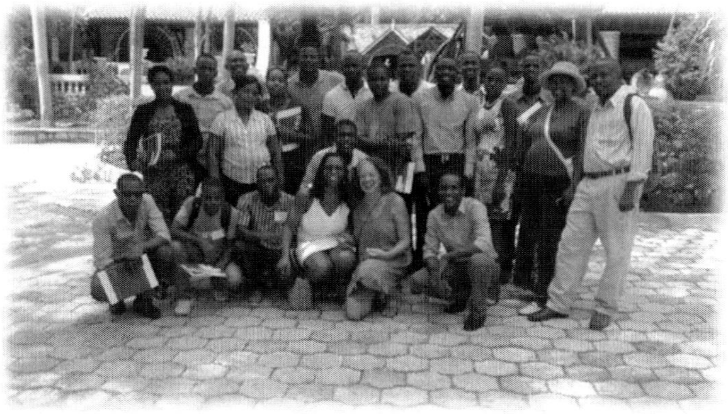

CONCLUSION

The Mental Health Training Program is designed to provide intensive psycho-educational training to health professionals, teachers, and community leaders on the signs, risk factors, and symptoms associated with various mental illnesses among children, adolescents, and adults; enhance providers' understanding of the impact of mental illness on individuals' physical, social and emotional development; and equip program participants with the knowledge that will enable them to better support individuals who are coping with mental illness. The training program is grounded in a community empowerment framework with objectives aimed at increasing capacity and sustainability of mental health treatment, providing training to diverse professionals and community members, and supporting ongoing efforts through a train the trainer model. As a capacity-building initiative, the HMHTP has built-in provisions to ensure that selected groups of trainers will continue to interact in meaningful ways by establishing a support system that can enhance their skills and capacity to provide mental health training to other providers, teachers, and community leaders in their respective communities.

REFERENCES

Albee, G. W. (1996). Revolutions and counterrevolutions in prevention. *American Psychologist, 51*(11), 1130-1133.

Colin, J. M., & Paperwalla, G. (1996). Haitians. In J. G. Lipson, S. L. Dibble, & P. A. Minarik (Eds.), *Culture and nursing care: A pocket guide* (pp. 139-154). San Francisco, CA: University of California, San Francisco Nursing Press. Cowen, E. (1991).

Cowen, E. (1994). The enhancement of psychological wellness: Challenges and opportunities. *American Journal of Community Psychology, 22*, 149-179.

Cowen, E. L. (1996). The ontogenesis of primary prevention: Lengthy strides and stubbed toes. *American Journal of Community Psychology,* 24,235-249.

Dunst, C. J., Trivette, C. M., & Thompson, R. (1990). Supporting and strengthening family functioning: Toward a congruence between principles and practice. *Prevention in the Human Services, 9*(1), 19-43.

Epp, H.T. 1988. Way of the migrant herds: Dual dispersion strategy among bison. *Plains Anthropologist* 33:309-20.

Miller, N. L. (2000). Haitian ethnomedical systems and biomedical practitioners: Directions for clinicians. Journal of Transcultural Nursing, 11, 204-11.

Munoz, R. E., Mrazek, P. J., & Haggerty, R. J. (1996). Institute of Medicine report on prevention of mental disorders: Summary and commentary. *American Psychologist, 51*, 1116-1122.

Nicolas, G., Arntz, D., Hirsch, B., & Schmiedigen, A. (2009). Cultural adaptation of a group treatment for Haitian American adolescents. *Professional Psychology: Research and Practice*, *40*(4), 378–384.

Nicolas, G., DeSilva, A. M., & Grey, K. S., & Gonzalez-Eastep, D. (2006). Using a multicultural lens to understand illnesses among Haitians living in America. *Professional Psychology: Research and Practice, 37*(6), 702-707.

Nicolas, G., DeSilva, A. M., Houlahan, S., & Beltrame, C. (2009). Culturally authentic scaling approach: A multi-step method for culturally adapting measures for use with ethnic minority and immigrant youths. *Journal of Youth Development, 4*(1), 81-95.

Pan American Health Organization (PAHO), Health in the Americas (2007). Washington, DC: PAHO, 2007, 425- 744 pp.

Prilleltensky, I. (1994). *The morals and politics of psychological discourse and the status quo*. Albany, NY: University of New York Press.

Rickel, A. U., & Becker, E. (1997). Keeping children from harm's way: How national policy affects psychological development. Washington, DC: American Psychological Association.

Trickett, P.K., Allen, L., Schellenbach, C.J. and Zigler, E.F. (1998) Integrating and Advancing the Knowledge Base About Violence Against Children: Implications for Intervention and Prevention. In P.K. Trickett and C.J. Schellenbach (Eds.) *Violence Against Children in the Family and the Community* (pp 419-437) Washington, DC: American Psychological Association.

Tucker CM, Herman KC, Ferdinand LA, Beato C, Adams D, Cooper L. (2007). Providing culturally sensitive healthcare: A formative model. *The Counseling Psychologist*, 35:679–705. doi: 10.1177/0011000007301689.

Watters, E. (2010). *Crazy like us: The globalization of the American psyche.* New York, NY: Free Press.

World Health Organization and UNICEF (1978). Primary Health Care: Report of the International Conference on Primary Health Care. Alma-Ata USSR. 6–12 September, 1978. Geneva: WHO.

Chapter 3

GUIDING PRINCIPLES FOR THE HAITI MENTAL HEALTH TRAINING PROGRAM

"More often, culture bears on whether people even seek help in the first place, what types of help they seek, what types of coping styles and social supports they have, and how much stigma they attach to mental illness. Culture also influences the meanings that people impart to their illness."

Culture Counts: The Influence of Culture and Society on Mental Health
A Supplement to Mental Health: A Report of the Surgeon General

INTRODUCTION

Low- and middle-income countries (LMICs) are disproportionately affected by the global burden of mental disorders (World Health Organization [WHO], 2001). While an estimated 450 million people are living with a mental illness around the world, close to 85% of those residing in LMICs do not have access to adequate mental health services (WHO, 2011). There are several contributing factors, including poverty, entrenched stigmas about mental illness, poverty, a lack of awareness or acknowledgement of mental health as a health care priority, limited infrastructure and financial resources, and a scarcity of mental health workers with the proper training and skills necessary to alleviate mental suffering among those afflicted with psychiatric disorders (Kutcher, Chehil, Cash, & Millar, 2005; Lund et al., 2010, 2011; Saraceno et al., 2007). As more culturally-sensitive training programs are needed to enhance the existing workforce capacity and reduce mental health disparities on a global level, it is imperative that such programs be grounded in theory and informed by evidence-based clinical practices and interventions that can promote mental health in low- and middle-income regions. Moreover, there needs to be a strong emphasis on active community engagement and participation as well as building and sustaining mental health capacity in these settings.

Research has shown that mental health programs that focus on training lay workers in low resource communities can contribute significantly to improved health and mental health outcomes in LMICs (Murray et al., 2011). As the need to increase capacity in these settings continues to rise, global mental health practitioners are pressed to identify, develop, and implement sustainable training programs and counseling intervention models, in particular those that can be adapted in other communities and countries throughout the world. One such model is the *Haiti Mental Health Training Program*, which has been used in various settings throughout the country for more than two decades. In this chapter, we describe the seven core principles that have guided the development of mental health capacity-building initiatives in Haiti. The chapter begins with a brief overview of the goals and objectives of the training model, followed by a description of the community empowerment framework upon which the model is based. The seven core principles of the *Haiti Mental Health Training Program* serve as the foundation for creating and sustaining community-based, culturally-oriented mental training programs in low and middle-income countries.

THE HAITI MENTAL HEALTH TRAINING PROGRAM

A detailed description of the Haiti Mental Health Training Program (HMHTP) is provided in Chapter 4. As such, only an overview of the program is provided here in order to fully understand the ways that the principles are infused throughout the training program. The HMHTP aims to:

(1) Provide intensive psycho-educational training to medical providers, teachers, community leaders, and other stakeholders on the signs, risk factors, and symptoms associated with various mental illnesses among Haitian children, adolescents, and adults;
(2) Enhance participants' awareness and understanding of the impact of mental illness on the social, emotional, and psychological well-being of Haitian individuals and families; and

(3) Equip program participants with the knowledge and skills to enable them to better serve and support members of their communities.

Inherent in the HMHTP is a "train-the-trainer" capacity-building model that has been applied successfully in various settings in Haiti, including schools, hospitals, and community-based organizations. The HMHTP is grounded in a community empowerment and sustainability framework that seeks to meet the following key objectives:

- Increase capacity and sustainability of mental health services in Haiti by training health professionals, teachers, religious leaders, and community members in psychosocial programming and implementation that is grounded in Haitian culture.
- Train health professionals, teachers, religious leaders, and community laypersons to recognize symptoms of psychological distress in individuals across different age groups and genders.
- Prepare health professionals, teachers, religious leaders, and community leaders to become trainers on how to conduct workshops with other groups in their respective communities.
- Utilize a "train-the-trainer" model to increase community awareness about mental health and mental illness, and ways of seeking services for these issues.

The HMHTP, which has been developed, implemented, and evaluated in Haiti over the past 20 years, is guided by the following seven core principles:

(1) Developing In-Country Partnerships,
(2) Enhancing Cultural Knowledge,
(3) Conducting a Community Needs Assessment,
(4) Selecting a Culturally Relevant Team,
(5) Creating a Culturally Relevant Curriculum,
(6) Conducting a Program Evaluation, and
(7) Building Local Capacity (see Figure 1).

The seven core principles of the HMHTP, which are based on guidelines provided by the World Health Organization (see Table 1), are described in further details below.

Table 1. 10 principles for integrating mental health into primary care

1.	The integration of mental health into policy and plans.
2.	Advocacy to address attitudes and behaviors towards mental health. (various sectors)
3.	Adequate (pre-service and/or in-service) training of primary care workers
4.	Primary care tasks must be limited and doable
5.	Specialist mental health professionals and facilities must be available to support primary care whether by referral or in collaborative models such as supervision.
6.	Access to essential psychotropic medications in primary care
7.	A commitment to integration as a process, not an event, which takes time and may occur over a number of years or a series of developments.
8.	A mental health service coordinator to oversee integration and foster effectiveness.
9.	Collaboration with other government non-health sectors, nongovernmental organizations, village and community health workers, and volunteers
10.	Financial and human resources are needed

(Adapted from World Health Organization and World Organization of Family Doctors Integrating mental health into primary care: A global perspective)

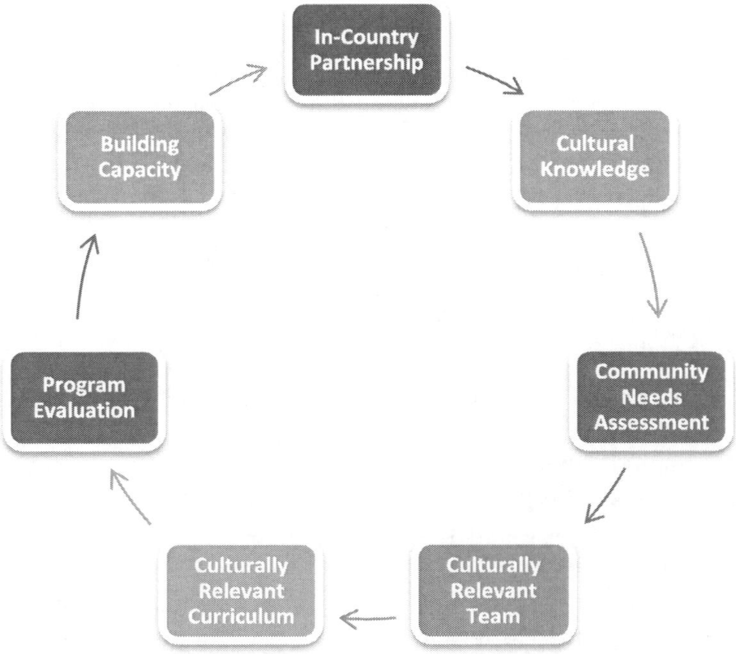

Figure 1. Seven Guiding Principles of the Mental Health Training Program in Haiti.

SEVEN CORE PRINCIPLES OF THE HAITI MENTAL HEALTH TRAINING PROGRAM

Principle 1: Developing In-Country Partnerships

Community participation and engagement are key components in the successful development and implementation of health promotion initiatives, psychoeducational interventions, and mental health training programs locally and across the globe (Palmer-Wackerly, Krok, Dailey, Kight, & Krieger, 2014). Community engagement is defined as "the process of working collaboratively with and through groups of people affiliated by geographic proximity, special interest, or similar situations to address issues affecting the well-being of those people" (Centers for Disease Control and Prevention, 1997, p. 9). Based on a report published by the Clinical and Translational Science Awards Consortium, "meaningful community participation [must extend] beyond physical involvement to include generation of ideas, contributions to decision making, and sharing of responsibility" (2011, p. 13).

It is well documented that active community engagement can yield significant benefits for all parties involved (Anderson et al., 2014; Roussos & Fawcett, 2000; Trickett et al., 2011). One reason is that community members who are actively involved in program development and implementation are more likely to remain engaged and stay motivated when their voices and needs are acknowledged, represented, and valued (Palmer-Wackerly et al., 2014). Additionally, engaging community stakeholders can facilitate trusting relationships between partner agencies, which can then improve communication, strengthen long-term collaborations, and build community capacity and sustainability (Anderson et al., 2014; Shore, 2006; Wallerstein, 2002).

Given the numerous benefits of active community engagement, researchers and practitioners working in LMICs must not only be cognizant of the unique needs of a community and its cultural nuances, but must also establish partnerships with local individuals and organizations prior to the development and implementation of programs. For mental health programs to be created and embedded successfully in international settings, partnerships with local government and key grassroots organizations are necessary. In Haiti, the success of the HMHTP can be attributed to the strong collaboration that emerged among several organizations and stakeholders who had a deep and rich understanding of the targeted communities as well as the needs of local consumers. These partnerships were forged between a Haiti-based team and a U.S.-based team during the early phase of the training program and remained in place throughout the development and implementation of the program.

The Haiti-based team was comprised of stakeholders (e.g., medical providers, teachers, religious and spiritual leaders, public officials, lay people) who were actively involved with the community. Members of the Haiti-based team were instrumental in providing consultation and on-going guidance to the U.S.-based team throughout the development and implementation phases of the program. Thus, the partnership was a direct response to the goals articulated by leaders and community members who resided in the different regions of the country and who were knowledgeable about the current needs of the local communities.

The U.S.-based team included the program developer, Dr. Nicolas who is a member of the Haitian Diaspora and a Haitian psychologist who was born in Haiti and completed her post-secondary education in the U.S. where she currently resides; health professionals of Haitian descent who were living in the Diaspora; and university researchers who worked in Haiti on issues related to health and mental health care. Many of these individuals also served as the initial team of trainers who became actively engaged in implementing the program in Haiti. This was an important component of the HMHTP, given that members of the Haitian Diaspora would already have some familiarity with the basics of social and professional interactions in Haiti. The U.S.-based team members and trainers included doctors, nurses, psychologists, and psychiatrists.

The U.S.-based team of researchers and health professionals worked in close collaboration with the Haiti-based team in order to gain perspectives on the current needs of the local community and to draw on existing resources. Given that stakeholders are often well acquainted with the needs of their community, culture, language, and norms and practices, they possess a richer understanding of the strategies that are most useful for engaging with the community and mechanisms that are most effective in implementing sustainable programs in the region. Thus, both professionals and community leaders were instrumental in identifying the appropriate fit for the development of the program, due to their familiarity with the overall landscape of the infrastructure, healthcare, and educational systems in Haiti.

Haiti-based partners were also responsible for maintaining the logistical aspects of the program. For example, each region had a local project manager or program assistant that was based in Haiti and represented a health care or educational establishment. Their responsibilities included ensuring logistical needs; communicating with doctors, nurses, teachers, and other stakeholders; coordinating community outreach efforts; organizing meetings among the local team members; and assisting with the mental health training program sessions.

As highlighted by our work with the HMHTP, in-country partnerships should reflect a collaborative relationship between teams in both countries (one local and one foreign) that comprise members who are either from the country of interest or are familiar with the country of interest in a meaningful way (e.g., having worked with members of its Diaspora, having visited or lived in the country for a period of time, being familiar with its history, etc.). In considering partnering with in-country organizations, it is best to select those that are already working with the target population in the community and are highly knowledgeable of the local needs of the population.

Principle 2: Enhancing Cultural Knowledge

In addition to building strong in-country partnerships, individuals who seek to engage in capacity-building initiatives in LMICs need to develop an understanding of the cultural norms and practices of the community of interest and how the community's cultural beliefs and values may affect such notions as meaning making and power sharing. In essence, such individuals must engage in an active process of becoming more culturally competent.

The concept of cultural competency has been widely studied in the literature (American Psychological Association, 2003; Stuart, 2004; Sue, Arredondo, & McDavis, 1992). It refers to the attitudes, awareness, knowledge, and skills that educators, practitioners, and researchers need to possess in order to provide quality services to individuals and groups from culturally diverse backgrounds (Sue & Sue, 2012). The need for cultural competency is even more pronounced when one is engaged in cross-cultural research and interventions, or program development and implementation on an international level.

Cultural competency may be demonstrated in several ways. First and foremost, researchers and practitioners working in international settings need to establish in-country partnerships with community leaders and representatives who possess a broad range of knowledge, experience, and expertise of the local area. As learners, they should acquire an intimate understanding of the local community prior to engaging in any outreach efforts or direct engagement in the country of interest. By seeking collaborations with, and consultation from, knowledgeable stakeholders, practitioners will gain an increased awareness and knowledge of the history and cultural context in which they will subsequently work. Furthermore, it is critical that practitioners engage in a process of self-education through immersion experiences, supplemented by information gathered from current literature and other resources that will foster a more intimate knowledge of the local context. This exploration/education process should also include other persons who would work on the project, in advance of outreach-based activities. Self-education through pre-travel and other forms of research will enable the practitioner to determine the type of staffing that may be needed in terms of both resources and fit.

For the Haiti program, the Project Investigator (Dr. Nicolas), first made frequent trips to the communities of interest. Despite having been born in the country, Dr. Nicolas sought to gain a better understanding of the local culture (for each region included in the project), including its unique history, needs, values, belief systems, and practices through group conversations, community forums, and frequent visits to the local region. It is erroneous to assume that because someone has visited or is originally from a country, s/he is adequately familiar with the culture and, as a result, does not need to acquire additional knowledge about that particular community. More training on the values and mores of the local context in which the programs will be implemented is often necessary. For example, by spending time in the local community as learners, the leaders of the HMHTP were able to gain greater insight and familiarity with the linguistic nuances that varied across the country, including proverbs, jokes, and folk tales. These materials, in turn, were subsequently included in the training manual used for the program. Thus, the manual was reflective of the local community in which the program was being implemented.

Additionally, members of the U.S.-based team were exposed to characteristics of the community of which residents were proud, and for which the community was known. Through this process of active engagement and direct immersion, team members were invited to meet with both key community stakeholders and local residents. For example, Dr. Nicolas met with mayors and the heads of the local hospital and school district as part of the initial planning process. She also went to local markets and had opportunities to become familiar with the needs, resources, and other nuances of the community of interest.

As a result, the staff that was selected for the project in the northern part of Haiti (i.e., Cap-Haïtien) was very different from the staff that was chosen to work in the southern part of the country (i.e., Petit-Goâve). Pre-travel and self-education also served as the impetus for not preparing all curriculum materials in advance. Although the project had manuals, the team soon learned that many of the manuals inadequately represented the local context. Thus, changes were made to the curriculum as time went by and additional information about the local community was acquired. The team only printed manuals on a session-by-session and region-by-region basis rather than in bulk and in advance of the training program.

In sum, the essence of the second principle—enhancing cultural knowledge—is for global mental health practitioners and researchers to remain open and curious as learners, to be culturally sensitive, and to shed preconceived notions or stereotypes that are not grounded in actual in-country immersion experiences, education, and information gathering activities (e.g., through pre-travel, reading of existing literature, etc.) relevant to the specific community in which they plan to conduct research, training, and counseling interventions.

Principle 3: Conducting a Community Needs Assessment

Given the unique needs of each community, once in-country partnerships are established, the next logical step is to engage in a community needs assessment to determine the types of services or programs that are needed for a particular group, assess the nature and causes of those needs, and develop a feasible action plan. A needs assessment is defined as "a systematic approach to identifying social problems, determining their extent, and accurately defining the target population to be served and the nature of their service needs" (Rossi, Lipsey, & Freeman, 1999, p. 119).

Community needs assessments are often conducted to generate ideas and document perceptions on important issues, gather preliminary data from key informants, guide decision-making processes, establish priorities for allocating resources towards meeting the specific needs of a community or group, and evaluate program outcomes. They require a step-by-step approach, which may include an exploration phase where a particular problem or concern is identified; a data gathering and analysis phase to identify community assets and resources as well as define the need for specific programs, interventions, or services; and a decision-making phase to prioritize needs, propose alternative solutions, and develop and implement a feasible action plan (Office of Migrant Education, 2001). Thus, effective community needs assessments must be designed and carried out in conjunction with key stakeholders (University of Kansas Work Group for Community Health and Development, 2015). Moreover, they need to incorporate a variety of tools, such as focus groups, community forums, listening sessions, interviews, field surveys, and the use of existing data that can best inform program development and implementation strategies.

The community needs assessments that were conducted as part of the HMHTP were largely informed by culturally oriented, participatory approaches to community engagement and capacity building. First, meetings were held with key stakeholders to gain an understanding of the community, region, and setting. For example, in Cap-Haïtien, the U.S.-based team met with the head of the largest hospital system in the region, Dr. Coq, to learn more about the hospital, its history, current programs, and activities. Several meetings were also held with the leaders of the various departments within the hospital, the director of the school of nursing, and the representative from the Ministry of Health in the region. In contrast, in Arcahaie (another region in Haiti), the team met with the elected mayor to get a better sense of the region, interventions and programs that were happening in the region, current needs of the community, and his perspectives on the proposed project. Subsequently, the mayor facilitated a number of face-to-face meetings with school principals and teachers in the region to discuss the scope of the project, gauge their interest in collaborating on the project, schedule school visits to obtain a better sense of the context in which the teachers were teaching, and gain a greater understanding of the training that teachers had received about mental health and the mental health needs of Haitian children, adolescents, and families.

Additionally, the U.S.-based team met with other local organizations to learn about their community-focused initiatives and to ensure that services would not be duplicated. Throughout the needs assessment process, team members compiled reading materials on the targeted area, met with residents, and conducted focus groups to capture the larger issues in the community, their current needs, and their recommendations for the best ways to address those issues.

Clearly, there are numerous reasons for conducting a comprehensive community needs assessment prior to implementing services and programs in LMICs. Information and data that are gathered, as well as the relationships that are formed during the needs assessment, will inform intervention strategies that are more culturally sound, improve community buy-in, enhance communication among partner organizations, and ensure sustainability of the project in the targeted community.

Principle 4: Selecting a Culturally Relevant Team

As discussed earlier in this chapter, researchers and practitioners need first and foremost to develop cultural knowledge of the region where they plan to work and acquire a firm understanding of the cultural values, belief systems, and practices of their targeted groups. These are essential components of in-country partnerships and central aspects of successful international projects. For the HMHTP, it was critical to plan and schedule meetings (in person or remotely) on a regular basis between the Haiti- and U.S.-based teams to clarify roles and responsibilities for each team, and to discuss the project and how it would be implemented. These meetings also assisted team members in becoming better acquainted with the cultural context, and in allowing issues such as language and gender differences to be explored and addressed beforehand. In order to be effective with our programs, it was important to ensure that the in-country staff and the U.S-based staff worked in continued collaboration. This facilitated a respectful and supportive environment where mutual learning could occur.

U.S.-Based Team

A prerequisite for the U.S.-based staff was that they would have adequate background in the Haitian culture and language to allow for easier communication to occur between the two teams. As such, the Haiti-based staff could hold U.S.-based staff accountable and provide a source of feedback regarding cultural nuances as well as logistics specific to the context. The team consisted of Haitian mental health professionals (i.e., psychologist, psychiatrists, social workers, and psychiatric nurses) who were born and raised in Haiti and immigrated to the U.S. in their late teens or adulthood. The team was selected based on their mental health background, linguistic abilities, familiarity with the culture, and ability to commit to several trips annually to Haiti for the project over the course of several years. Once team members were selected, conference calls were scheduled to provide an orientation to the program, get connected with each other, and create a work plan. Additionally, prior to the first trip to Haiti, the team received training on the curriculum and the community in which the program would be implemented.

Haiti-Based Team

The in-country partnership consisted of identifying an individual who would lead the program in Haiti; this individual also took responsibility for identifying others who could serve as members of the Haiti-based team for the program. Selection of team members depended on the focus of the project. For example, the community mental health project in Petit-Goâve consisted of team members from various backgrounds such as psychology students, communication specialists, and religious and community leaders. However, team members for the program focusing on integrating mental health into primary care settings in Cap-Haïtien consisted mainly of a family physician, a psychologist, social worker, and a nurse practitioner. Meetings similar to those held with the U.S.-based team were also conducted to orient the local team about the purpose and objectives of the program.

Coming Together

Prior to implementing the project, the two teams met in Haiti to familiarize themselves with one another, review program logistics, and obtain additional training on the curriculum. These meetings were crucial in facilitating team building and cohesion, enhancing communication, and promoting trust among group members. It was a unique opportunity for the teams to also learn from each other about ways to more effectively deliver the curriculum as well as develop a better understanding of each other's styles.

A good example of a teachable moment for the U.S.-based team came during the implementation of the program in Cap-Haïtien. When the U.S.-based team learned that some program participants would have a daily commute of more than two hours to attend the week-long training, they recommended that hotel accommodations be made for the Haiti-based team to reside closer to the project site during the monthly training sessions. The trainees and trainers in Haiti, however, declined the offer and reported that the stay would displace them from their families, even if it was only for one week. Our own U.S.-based cultural framework led us to believe that an hour-long commute each way would be a hassle that could easily be eliminated with a hotel stay; however, we quickly learned from the Haiti-based trainers that it was more important for them to be with their families on a daily basis than to have a shorter commute. By interfacing with the in-country team on the various aspects of the program development and implementation, we realized that this different response had much to do with the cultural values and customs in Haiti. Such reciprocal learning was instrumental in ensuring that we developed an effective working relationship with each other.

Language

Taking into account which language would be used for the training program was also critical. In Haiti, French is perceived as the language of the educated or informed individual. With this knowledge, program leaders engaged in on-going discourse with the in-country team to address the reality that the majority of the Haitian community speaks Haitian Creole or Kreyòl. While training materials were made available in both French and Haitian Kreyòl, over time, program participants embraced the shift from speaking French (or showing preference for the French manuals) to speaking Kreyòl and learning the concepts using the Kreyòl language manuals. They also recognized the important role of the native language in the history of the country and the region where the program was being implemented. Encouraging such a shift involved a delicate balance that did not entail imposing an outsider's view, but rather carefully using cultural knowledge and awareness of nuances to recognize important dynamics that could compromise the effectiveness of reaching the overall goals of the program and to foster a shift using a culturally respectful approach.

Gender

Similar to language, gender is an important construct to which practitioners and researchers need to attend. In our work in Haiti, participants subscribed to traditional gender and status roles that were intricately interrelated. For instance, during community meetings, doctors (who were predominantly males) initially spoke up more, while nurses (who were mostly females) hesitated to speak and felt like their voices were not or could not be heard. Over several weeks, the trainers worked collaboratively to create a context where all voices would be heard and respected, and where nurses would feel valued enough to share their thoughts and input. This paradigm shift was emphasized and incorporated into every level of the training of trainers who themselves had become more aware of gender dynamics through their own participation as trainees, making the shift more sustainable over time. For example, groups were created with both doctors and nurses, rather than having groups isolated by profession, and trainers intentionally invited a variety of perspectives.

As the program evolved, nurses began to share with doctors important information about their profession, such as the level of interaction that they had with patients. The process became a fruitful learning experience and allowed for community building and group cohesion among the team members. Without an understanding and awareness of the nuances of the Haitian healthcare system and culture, it would have been challenging to identify such potentially problematic dynamics and to work to change them over time in a sensitive and strategic manner.

Principle 5: Creating a Culturally-Relevant Curriculum

One may envision the process of creating a culturally-relevant mental health curriculum as an inverted triangle or funnel. In order to develop such a curriculum, it is best to start at the broad general level, with what is already known, and then review in detail what is relevant (and may remain as is), and what will need to be modified, deleted, or added. This revision process should be facilitated by a dialogue with the key participants in the country of interest who can provide insight and input into what is culturally valid and relevant.

Our program curriculum began with covering mental health issues generally and then more specifically by incorporating culturally-bound syndromes and disorders, and providing examples of how they are manifested in Haiti. To explain further, we first looked at the research on global mental health disorders. Then we reviewed the predominant mental health issues among ethnically diverse populations, especially among Black individuals. This enabled us to identify which disorders were more prevalent for these particular groups. The most commonly occurring disorders were depression, anxiety, trauma, and grief. We then added coping because we deemed it equally important to highlight the natural internal resources upon which people rely in their everyday life. In order to make the curriculum culturally relevant, we sought guidance from psychologists, psychiatrists, social workers, nurses, and religious and spiritual leaders in Haiti. In particular, we wanted to make sure that the labels that we were using were reflective of the Haitian culture and language. For example, in Haiti there is no Kreyòl word for the English word *Anxiety*. Thus, it was important for us to conduct research to understand the label that is often used in Haitian culture/language to refer to the cluster of symptoms that mirror Anxiety. Through such investigation, we learned of the phrase "kè sou biskèt" (translated to English, it means fluttering heart). We also gained insight on the specific warning signs and risk factors for both children and adults for each of the identified disorders and captured common idioms of distress in the targeted community.

While the basics of the curriculum remained the same, each program had different versions of the training booklet to ensure that the curriculum maintained its cultural relevance for the different regions in Haiti. As such, program participants contributed significantly to the continuous revision of the content of the training manual. In so doing, participants were both students and experts in developing the program. It was important for the manuals to serve as working documents that were updated as new cultural knowledge became available. During each training session, for instance, program participants would address key issues that were relevant to the contents of an upcoming session. As we learned of components that were not relevant, we removed the information from the manual, and updated the curriculum with newly acquired information. To ensure that this was maintained on an on-going basis, training manuals were printed just prior to each week-long training session. This allowed us to include culturally-specific symptomology and other key information that emerged through discussions of the previous week's training. The manual therefore served as a live, dynamic document, which was co-created by participants and trainers/program developers. The final result is a set of training manuals that have now been translated into three languages—English, French, and Kreyòl.

Principle 6: Conducting a Program Evaluation

The specific components of the program evaluation that accompanied the Haiti Mental Health Training Program are presented in a separate section of this monograph. In this chapter, we will define program evaluation, provide a brief overview of the HMHTP evaluation process, and address the relevance of program evaluations in sustaining mental health training programs in low- and middle-income countries.

Program evaluation refers to "the use of social research procedures to systematically investigate the effectiveness of programs or services" (Rossi et al., 1999, p. 4). A program evaluation may be conducted for the purpose of program improvement, accountability, acquisition of new knowledge, and informed policies and best practices. Program evaluations typically involve the assessment of one or more of five program domains: (1) determining the need for a program or service, (2) evaluating the design of a program or service, (3) assessing the implementation of a program or service, (4) measuring program outcomes, and (5) evaluating the efficiency of a program or service (Rossi et al., 1999).

The two most common types of program evaluation are process or formative evaluation and outcome or summative evaluation. Process/formative evaluation refers to the assessment of a program's components to determine whether the services that are being implemented will result in the desired outcomes. Outcome/summative evaluation assesses the extent to which a program has met its stated goals and objectives (Rossi et al., 2004).

While numerous evidence-informed program evaluation models have been cited in the literature (e.g., Centers for Disease Control & Prevention, 1999;

Milstein & Wetherall, 2000), there is a dearth of guidelines and resources for evaluating programs and services in LMICs specifically. Milstein and Wetherall (2000) proposed a 6-step framework that summarizes in a logical manner the main components of a program evaluation. They include engaging stakeholders, describing the program, focusing the evaluation design, gathering credible evidence from multiple sources, justifying findings and conclusions, and sharing lessons learned. Such a framework model may be modified and tailored to an individual community's unique context and needs.

For the HMHTP, the program evaluation was conducted at multiple levels. There was a pre-assessment, which was used to gather preliminary information about participants' knowledge and understanding of mental health-related concepts. A demographic questionnaire was utilized for data collection purposes. Additionally, throughout the course of the training, there were ongoing group activities, which allowed participants to provide immediate input into the content of the training materials, the implementation process, group dynamics, and the overall structure of the training program.

Lastly, at the end of the weekly training program, a post-assessment was conducted. It included an exam that measured participants' knowledge and understanding of the topic discussed during the training session, a group presentation given by program participants, and participants' verbal and written feedback regarding their training experience. Those strategies were used intentionally to ensure active stakeholder engagement, gather both quantitative and qualitative data from program participants, identify potential challenges and opportunities, and incorporate lessons learned and recommendations into future training programs. This information was then fed back to the local team to assist them in the implementation of the program.

In sum, program evaluation is essential in the development and implementation of community-based interventions and services. In low- and middle-income settings where resources are scarce, the process of program evaluation is urgently needed to ensure program functioning and success, ongoing improvement, and sustainability.

Principle 7: Building Community Capacity – "Train-the-Trainer" Model

Capacity building generally refers to a process aimed at increasing the skills, infrastructure, and resources of individuals, organizations, and communities (Taveras et al., 2007). One of the key elements of implementing programs and services in international settings is ensuring that the programs are sustainable over time. While there are many ways of maintaining sustainability, one of the most successful aspects of the HMHTP was the "train-the-trainer" model, which was built into the program from its inception.

A review of the literature indicates that the train-the-trainer (TTT) approach is a strategy that has been widely used in a variety of contexts and for numerous purposes, including education, prevention, and building training capacity in community-based settings (Howze, Auld, Woodhouse, Gershick, & Livingood, 2009; Orfaly, Frances, Campbell, Whittemore, Joly, & Koh, 2005; Pearse et al., 2012; Tobias, Downes, Eddens, & Ruiz, 2012). TTT models typically involve the dissemination of knowledge, information, and skills delivered by professionals to groups of trainers (e.g., volunteers, health care providers, faith-based and community leaders, military personnel, first responders, lay persons) who, in turn, share those skills and knowledge with others in their respective communities (Connell, Holmes, Voelkl, & Bazaar, 2002).

There are numerous benefits to utilizing TTT models. First, program leaders can provide intensive training to a small number of individuals who can then be responsible for organizing and facilitating future training workshops and group activities (Tobias et al., 2012). Second, qualified trainers can serve as cultural brokers due to their personal connections with members of their communities and, as a result, may engage in more effective outreach efforts (Tobias et al., 2012). Furthermore, as a capacity-building health promotion approach, TTT models can not only enhance the knowledge base at the local level and strengthen the capacity of communities with limited resources, but it can ensure program sustainability beyond the initial stages of program development and implementation.

For the HMHTP, at the end of each training session, between three and five participants were chosen as trainers for future sessions. The selection of trainers was done in a strategic but equitable manner. The participants were selected based on a number of factors, including their grasp of the training materials, ease in group interactions, and availability to facilitate future training sessions. Selected participants became co-facilitators with the U.S.-based teams and, ultimately, served as the next group of trainers once their training session was completed. A trainers' manual was developed to provide the trainers with step by step guidelines for implementation of the program.

This community capacity-building approach included designating a set number of days in which selected trainers were trained on the goals and objectives of the project, evaluating trainers' grasp of the materials, and ensuring trainers' readiness to lead subsequent training groups of new trainees in their entirety. As the program progressed, the U.S.-based team became consultants to the in-country teams, and was no longer needed to facilitate training sessions. It is important to have a plan in place for the transition to occur, and to establish a viable and appropriate communication channel that will serve as the link between the in-country (host) leaders and the U.S.-based team where questions and consultations can take place and additional resources can be shared based on different issues that may arise along the way.

CONCLUSION

This chapter provided an overview of the framework for the Mental Health Training Program in Haiti and the seven core principles that have guided the development and implementation of the HMHTP over the past two decades. Given the fact that the program has been implemented in various regions of Haiti for more than two decades, this is a model that can be adapted to address mental health needs and build workforce capacity in other low- and middle-income countries. As the research literature indicates, the needs for mental health services in these countries are great, but it is essential that researchers and practitioners do work that is sustainable, culturally informed, and relevant in order to be as effective as possible, minimize harm, and remain mindful of the impact that such programs can have on a local level.

REFERENCES

American Psychological Association. (2003). Guidelines on multicultural education, training, research, practice, and organizational change for psychologists. *American Psychologist, 58*, 377-402.

Anderson, F., Donkor, P., de Vries, R., Appiah-Denkyira, E., Dakpallah, G. F., Rominski, S., … Ayettey, S. (2014). Creating a charter of collaboration for international university partnerships: The Elmina Declaration for Human Resources for Health. *Academic Medicine: Journal of the Association of American Medical Colleges, 89*(8), 1125-1132.

Centers for Disease Control and Prevention. (1997). *Principles of community engagement.* Retrieved from http://www.atsdr.cdc.gov/ community engagement/.

Centers for Disease Control and Prevention. (1999). Framework for program evaluation in public health. *MMWR, 48*(No. RR-11). Retrieved from http://www.cdc.gov/mmwr/pdf/rr/rr4811.pdf.

Clinical and Translational Science Awards Consortium. (2011). *Principles of community engagement.* Washington, DC: Department of Health and Human Services, NIH Publication No. 11-7782. Retrieved from http://www.atsdr.cdc.gov/communityengagement/pdf/PCE_Report_508_FINAL.pdf.

Connell, C. M., Holmes, S. B., Voelkl, J. E., & Bazaar, H. R. (2002). Providing dementia outreach education to rural communities: Lessons learned from a train-the-trainer program. *Journal of Applied Gerontology,* 21(3), 294–313.

Howze, E. H., Auld, M. E., Woodhouse, L. D., Gershick, J., & Livingood, W. C. (2009). Building health promotion capacity in developing countries: Strategies from 60 years of experience in the United States. *Health Education & Behavior, 36*, 464–475.

Kutcher, S., Chehil, S., Cash, C., & Millar, J. (2005). A competencies-based mental health training model for health professionals in low and middle income countries. *World Psychiatry, 4*(3), 177-180.

Lund, C., De Silva, M., Plagerson, S., Cooper, S., Chisholm, D., Jishnu, D., ... Patel, V. (2011). Poverty and mental disorders: Breaking the cycle in low-income and middle-income countries. *The Lancet, 378(9801)*, 1502-1514.

Lund, C., Breen, A., Flisher, A., Kakuma, R., Corrigall, J., Joska, J., ... Patel, V. (2010). Poverty and common mental disorders in low and middle income countries: A systematic review. *Social Science & Medicine, 71*(3), 517-528.

Milstein, B., & Wetherall, S. (2000). A framework featuring steps and standards for program evaluation. *Health Promotion Practice, 1*(3), 221-228.

Murray, L. K., Dorsey, S., Bolton, P., Jordans, M. J. D., Rahman, A., Bass, J., & Verdeli, H. (2011). Building capacity in mental health interventions in low resource countries: An apprenticeship model for training local providers. *International Journal of Mental Health Systems, 5*(30), 1-12.

Office of Migrant Education. (2001). *Comprehensive needs assessment.* Retrieved from http://www2.ed.gov/admins/lead/account/compneedsassessment.pdf.

Orfaly, R. A., Frances, J. C., Campbell, P., Whittemore, B., Joly, B., & Koh, H. (2005). Train-the-trainer as an educational model in public health preparedness. *Journal of Public Health Management and Practice*, S123–S127.

Palmer-Wackerly, A. L., Krok, J. L., Dailey, P. M., Kight, L., & Krieger, J. L. (2014). Community engagement as a process and an outcome of developing culturally grounded health communication interventions: An example from the DECIDE Project. *American Journal of Community Psychology, 53*, 261-274.

Rossi, P., Lipsey, M., & Freeman, H. (1999). *Evaluation: A systematic approach* (6th ed.). Thousand Oaks, CA: Sage.

Roussos, S. T., & Fawcett, S. B. (2000). A review of collaborative partnerships as a strategy for improving community health. *Annual Review of Public Health, 21*, 369–402.

Saraceno, B., van Ommeren, M., Batniji, R., Cohen, A., Gureje, O., Mahoney, J., ... Underhill, C. (2007). Barriers to improvement of mental health services in low-income and middle-income countries. *Lancet, 370*, 1164-1174.

Shore, N. (2006). Re-conceptualizing the Belmont Report: A community-based participatory research perspective. *Journal of Community Practice, 14*(4), 5-26.

Stuart, R. B. (2004). Twelve practical suggestions for achieving multicultural competence. *Professional Psychology: Research & Practice, 35*(1), 3-9.

Sue, D. W., Arredondo, P., & McDavis, R. J. (1992). Multicultural counseling competencies and standards: A call to the profession. *Journal of Counseling & Development, 70*(4), 477-486.

Sue, D. W., & Sue, D. (2012). *Counseling the culturally diverse: Theory and practice* (6th ed.). New York, NY: John Wiley & Sons.

Taveras, S., Duncan, T., Gentry, D., Gilliam, A., Kimbrough, I., & Minaya, J. (2007). The evolution of the CDC HIV prevention capacity-building assistance initiative. *Journal of Public Health Management and Practice* (Suppl.), S8-15.

Tobias, C. R., Downes, A., Eddens, S., & Ruiz, J. (2012). Building blocks for peer success: Lessons learned from a train-the-trainer program. *AIDS Patient Care and STDs, 26*(1), 53-59.

Trickett, E. J., Beehler, S., Deutsch, C., Green, L. W., Hawe, P., McLeroy, K., et al. (2011). Advancing the science of community-level interventions. *American Journal of Public Health, 101*(8), 1410–1419. doi:10.2105/AJPH.2010.300113.

University of Kansas Work Group for Community Health and Development. (2015). *Community assessment, agenda setting, and choice of broad strategies*. Lawrence, KS: Community Tool Box. Retrieved from http://ctb.ku.edu/en/table-of-contents.

Wallerstein, N. (2002). Empowerment to reduce health disparities. *Scandinavian Journal of Public Health Supplement, 59*, 72-77.

World Health Organization. (2001). *The world health report 2001 – Mental health: New understanding, new hope.* Retrieved from http://www.who.int/whr/2001/media_centre/press_release/en/.

World Health Organization. (2011). *Global burden of mental disorders and the need for a comprehensive, coordinated response from health and social sectors at the country level*. Geneva, Switzerland: World Health Organization.

Chapter 4

LOCALS AS EXPERTS: BUILDING LOCAL PARTNERSHIPS INTERNATIONALLY

"The best partnerships aren't dependent on a mere common goal but on a shared path of equality, desire, and no small amount of passion."

Sarah MacLean

Currently, many international projects are implemented as a "helicopter like" approach with very little partnerships with in country organizations and thus often these programs are short lived. Chapter 3 outlined the guiding principles of the Haiti Mental Health Training Program. The first principle, Developing In-country Partnerships, is the foundational basis for the additional six principles. In order to successfully design, implement, and sustain a mental health-training program at the international level, you must develop deliberate partnerships and collaborations. A partnership is a purposeful collaboration of joint stakeholders who have a common purpose and end goal. Furthermore, an international partnership necessitates an understanding of culture, an emphasis on power-sharing, and an acknowledgement of local people as experts. In this chapter, we review important elements of international and cross-cultural partnerships and collaborations. We discuss the steps we have taken in building partnerships in Haiti as a guide for replication in any context. Furthermore, we provide key points for establishing and sustaining the partnerships you develop.

Overview of International and Cross-Cultural Partnership

As previously discussed, there is a lack of literature concerning international mental health partnerships with LMICs in the Caribbean. Nevertheless, several writers have documented international partnerships for building capacity in health, mental health, and education. The following literature provides some examples of successful processes and important lessons.

Zheng and colleagues (2001) describe a nursing partnership between the University of Michigan School of Nursing and Peking University in China. While recognizing the different cultural and sociopolitical contexts of the two universities, the partnership was formed based on global principles of the nursing profession. Faculty collaborations included scholarly exchanges of curricular material, joint research, faculty and student exchanges, and educational workshops. The authors share that success of the project was built upon "mutual respect, as well as common interests and goals" (Zheng et al., 2001, p.121). They also stress that patience is a vital component in that timelines can change and collaborative decision-making requires time and understanding. The authors reported that the Michigan and Peking partnership was mutually beneficial and required cross-cultural learning and understanding. An important lesson learned in that collaboration was that each step of the process required more time than planned. In order to successfully reach decisions with consensus, great patience and cultural understanding is required.

Sider (2014) describes a collaborative partnership for building leadership capacity among Haitian school leaders. The collaboration between Haitian and Canadian leaders involved using technology and the web to communicate and problem solve. This involved participants from both countries as co-mentors engaged in reciprocal learning (Sider, 2014). Evaluation of this Digital Mentoring Project brought out three major themes about the collaboration: collaboration and problem solving; adapted leadership practices; and local and cross-cultural learning. Sider highlights that through continuous collaborative contact, the Haitian leaders learned from each other and even partnered with one another to create and provide workshops for teachers. This example shows that the locals themselves can be valuable resources to one another. Emphasis must not be placed solely on what foreign partners can offer the low resourced country in which they are working.

The work of international partnerships involves a process of careful planning that is guided by theory, practice, and experience. Ogilvie, Allen, Laryea, & Opare (2003) applied the theoretical principles of empowerment and capacity building to better understand international partnerships. Ogilvie and colleagues describe a capacity building project between nursing faculty at the University of Ghana and the University of Alberta. Ogilvie and colleagues highlight that "building capacity in its broadest sense encompasses the development of physical, human, organizational, social, and cultural capital. All are important and all require attention in planning, implementing, and evaluating development projects" (Ogilvie et al., 2003, p.114). Additionally, empowerment theory posits that individuals and communities must not only perceive their power to enact changes but also to build or develop the knowledge, skills, and resources necessary to meet their set goals.

Ng and colleagues (2013) provides a documentation of mental health partnerships in low and middle income countries as part of the Asia-Pacific Community Mental Health Development Project (APCMHDP). Similar to Haiti, the Asia-Pacific region suffers from a mental health service gap. The APCMHDP detail ten guiding principles illustrated by examples of 17 participating countries that included the following best practices:

1. Identify key community mental health stakeholders;
2. Develop a common purpose and commitment;
3. Establish mutual respect between partners and appreciation of differences;
4. Develop good communication between partners;
5. Involve service users;
6. Involve families and caregivers;
7. Focus on a recovery model that promotes rehabilitation and social inclusion;
8. Include partners from both health and non-health sectors;
9. Engage in coordination and management of tasks between partners;
10. Have clear governance structures and accountability.

Overall, existing literature highlights the importance of mutuality in terms of respect and shared goals when building partnerships. It also illuminates the care and attention that must be paid to valuing the cross-cultural relationship. With this understanding we now will describe the partnerships built in Haiti for the Mental Health Training Program.

Key Attributes in Building Partnerships Internationally: Examples from the Haiti Project

When pursuing international partnerships, you need to first identify the stakeholders. Depending on the country where you are seeking collaborations, the systemic structures may vary. For example, in Haiti organizations providing mental health services are not widely available. Because of the stigma mental illness carries within the culture, the discussion of mental health primarily takes place with medical providers and spiritual or religious leaders. Therefore the development of a mental health training program also relies on less conventional partnerships. The first step in identifying the stakeholders must involve meeting with key informants. Meetings with key informants and stakeholders help to clarify community needs, goals and stakeholder commitments. The following section describes the stakeholders involved in the Haiti Mental Health Training program. Next we provide details of the process that we undertook in building local partnerships. Lastly, we outline key factors in maintaining a strong partnership.

Identifying Key Informants, Stakeholders, and Partners

Key informants can range from local people well-known in the community to elected officials or politicians. Whether you are invited in because of your expertise or you are seeking to offer your skills to a community, meeting with key informants serves several functions. Key informants have social capital. They will know the present needs of the community as well as the historical barriers. They also know the current and historical strengths and resources that might be available for the development of a successful project. Key informants are insiders and can facilitate access to information and connections to stakeholders. If the importance of their role is neglected or not respected, they can also create barriers to the success of your project. Key informants have power or influence. Building a trusting relationship with key informants is vital to the process of building local partnerships. Key informants have the respect of the stakeholders who may be leery of the intentions of outsiders seeking collaborations in their community.

Stakeholders are those community members who have an opportunity to benefit or potentially be harmed by the project being implemented. The impact of any project must be assessed for potential risks and benefits of relevant stakeholders. Among the identified stakeholders, you will find the partners required for building a sustainable team.

Elected Officials

Key informants, such as elected officials or politicians are stakeholders who have power and authorization, especially as especially as it's pertains to policy. It is important to respect the political structure of a community in which you wish to work and build partnerships. Even if there are assumptions of political corruption or instability within a community, you must respect the existing structure and learn the processes for establishing partnerships within that setting. Elected officials may help provide the framework and conditions under which the project will be allowed to move forward.

Formal Care Providers

The Mental Health Training Program included partnerships with medical providers. Medical providers are often a resource for people suffering from mental illness or distress. However, in the absence of trained psychiatrist and other mental health practitioners, doctors and nurses may lack the expertise to diagnose and treat mental health problems. Furthermore, they may not have a focus that includes promoting mental health and well-being as a part of their medical practice. In low and middle-income countries, those in need of mental health services may reach out to medical providers with somatic complaints stemming from mental illness, trauma, or distress. Medical providers are important stakeholders in promoting mental well-being and guiding patients with mental health concerns towards wellness.

As stakeholders, medical professionals are concerned with the overall well-being of the patients whom they serve. In cultures such as Haiti where mental illness is stigmatized, formal medical care can be sought from doctors and nurses without the fear of being labeled as mentally ill or "crazy". Medical professionals are appropriately poised to educate their consumers about mental illness as well as mental health and wellbeing. Consumers of health services trust their providers and are less resistant to following the advice of these professionals. Partnering with local health professionals can add to the credibility of international partners seeking to provide mental health training or services in a host country.

Informal Care Providers: Spiritual Leaders

Religious and spiritual leaders also serve as resources for treatment where gaps in mental health services exist. Although these leaders are not formally trained in health or mental health, there in-depth understanding of the mind-body relationship marks them as a critical resource for those who cannot access formal medical care. As respected members of the community, spiritual leaders are closely connected with individuals and families that may be in need. These leaders often possess knowledge of alternative medicines and herbs that can help calm symptoms of disease or distress.

Educators

Teachers and educational leaders have valued roles in the community, particularly among the poor. Education plays a vital role in economic and social mobility, thereby raising the respect for teachers within society. Teachers can be valuable stakeholders in promoting mental health and well-being. They are uniquely situated for the daily observation of children and adolescents. Teachers can become liaisons in educating families about mental illness and promoting mental health.

Community Leaders and Organizers

Community center directors and workers are examples of other important stakeholders and potential partners. Community organizers are those individuals and groups that are already mobilized within a community. Although their focus may be on other aspects of civic engagement, their ability to engage community members in action is essential to the successful application of a program. The skills of community organizers and leaders lie in their knowledge of the community being served, connections with individuals of influence, and trust of the local people.

Local Businesses-Private Sector

One might not think of local businesses as key stakeholders when undertaking an international mental health partnership program. However, the private sector businesses are valuable community members who have resources you will likely need. Local businesses should be explored for providing venues for trainings and meeting that will be convenient to local participants. Local hotels and restaurants will be needed for accommodations for international partners and program catering. Additionally, local businesses are a resource for cultural exploration and learning by the foreign staff and partners who will need to build understanding and awareness.

LESSONS FROM HAITI

The Mental Health Training Program is implemented with the full collaboration of local partners. The process and types of partnerships differed depending on the specific needs and focus of the communities. Details are provided for two regions in which the project was implemented in Haiti.

Mental Health Training Program with Health Professionals in Cap Haitien

Cap Haitien is Haiti's second largest city (population approximately 200,000) and has the nation's second largest public hospital, Hopital Universitaire Justinien (HUJ). The HUJ is the sole hospital serving Cap Haitien and is also the referral hospital for the entire Northern Health Department of Haiti, serving a population of 1 million people. The HUJ is an academic center affiliated with three medical schools in Haiti and a school of nursing which is located adjacent to the hospital. HUJ is a 250-bed facility and has the full range of medical services including family medicine, internal medicine, pediatrics, orthopedics, obstetrics and gynecology, general surgery, anesthesiology, orthopedics, otolaryngology and ophthalmology and a preventive/Public Health unit. The HUJ has 35 physicians and 100 nurses. The hospital has numerous international partners who are helping in areas of research, practice, and development of infrastructure. In addition to medical, surgical, and technical needs, identifying and treating mental health issues remains an area for growth in the region.

The Haiti Project is a long standing physician training program in HUJ organized by two faculty members from the University of Miami (UM). This existing collaboration between UM and HUJ facilitated further collaboration across disciplines. A member of the Haiti Project, initiated a conversation with the first author, subsequent to the 2010 Haiti earthquake. In the weeks and months after the earthquake, the physicians were seeing many patients with various physical health complaints for which no clinical explanations could be found. Dr. Nicolas, a psychologist and faculty member at University of Miami met with Dr. Vulcain to discuss the cases.

As discussed earlier in this chapter, an invitation by a key informant is only the first step in undergoing an international project. Dr. Nicolas assembled a team of people for a field visit to Cap Haitien to further assess the needs. The team met with the head of the hospital in addition to various other heads of departments. The team also met with the regional minister of health. These key stakeholder interviews concluded with the team compiling a report of what was learned. Dr. Nicolas met again with the head of the hospital and Dr. Vulcian to provide a summary of the findings and determine next steps. It was determined that a mental health training program would be beneficial to the hospital staff. The level of commitment to hosting trainings on mental health was assessed and an agreement reached.

Hosting the trainings was specifically defined with clear requirements of the stakeholders. These stakeholders, including the minister of health agreed to be present at every training. This meant that during a week-long training, they would be in attendance to welcome trainees on the first day and/or last day of the session. These key stakeholders would address the trainees as to who the U.S. based training team were in Cap Haitien. Although this may seem a small detail, it serves an important function. The participants in the training were made aware that the training team was invited by local stakeholders and were working in partnership. This created trust early on between the trainees and the U.S. based trainers.

Dr. Nicolas and her team scheduled another visit to Cap Haitian to gather data and gain understanding of cultural elements. Having implemented mental health training curricula in Haiti and elsewhere previously, Dr. Nicolas needed to change the training manual to reflect the culture of this specific region. They spent one week immersed in the local culture, learning the nuances of the dialect in order to assure a culturally appropriate curriculum. The curriculum was also regularly updated whenever the local trainers identified better ways of capturing a concept linguistically. As this is a train-the-trainer model, the local partners and trainers own the project. The international trainers then serve as consultants and supporters, visiting monthly as needed.

Mental Health Training Program with Teachers in Arcahaie

The mental health training program in Arcahaie developed in a similar fashion. Dr. Nicolas was invited by a friend to bring the training program to this region. Arcahaie is located about one hour outside of Haiti's capital city Port-au-Prince. Arcahaie is a historic city, boasting as the birthplace of the Haitian flag.

Being invited by a knowledgeable key informant and stakeholder is an honor that comes with great responsibility. Nevertheless, having one contact who is seeking your collaboration is insufficient for creating a sustainable mental health training program internationally. The key informant recognized the mental health needs in the community and the lack of mental health resources. There were no mental health clinics available in this region. Furthermore, those serving the community such as religious leaders, health professionals, public officials, and teachers had very little formal knowledge of mental illness or mental health and wellbeing.

Dr. Nicolas came to this region with her U.S. based team. They met with the Mayor of the city of Arcahaie as well as the mayor of St Marc, the neighboring city that is part of the Arcahaie region. The catalyst for seeking training on mental health was also a result of the 2010 earthquake. Stakeholders within the community were seeing trauma reactions among residents, but did not know how to address them. The public officials were chiefly concerned about the children in the community and how to help meet their emotional needs. Thus schools were seen as ideal partners in this endeavor.

The mayor of Arcahaie scheduled a meeting with all of the heads of schools in the region to meet with Dr. Nicolas and the team. Fifteen schools participated in the meeting from the plains to the mountains. They all agreed that a program was needed that could help them better understand and meet the needs of the youth in the community. This meeting allowed the heads of schools to formally agree to be partners in adopting the mental health training program. Their cooperation was vital to assuring that teachers will be given the leave time to participate in the training program.

Although the schools were principle stakeholders and important partners in the collaboration, there were many additional partnerships formed. Before undertaking the project, the team met with programs in the area such as Hope on a String. This is a program focusing on community development through music education. Another local program that was engaged for collaboration was Haiti Futur, which was new to the region and was developing smart boards for teachers. The Musée Ogier Fombrun also became a key partner. Located on a former sugar plantation in the Arcahaie region, Musée Ogier Fombrun contains Haitian artifacts that predate Columbus, from the Indian era to colonial times. Many of the training participants visit this museum for the first time during the mental health-training program. A key aspect of the culturally relevant mental health program is to recognize that history and legacy is a central component to talking about identity and self-esteem. The Barr Foundation was also an instrumental partner as it is a funding agency of programs in the region.

Local businesses can play important roles when undertaking international projects. For the Mental Health Training Program in Haiti local businesses were used to provide food and venues for trainings, accommodations for U.S. based training staff and partners, and cultural learning opportunities. Investigating local resources and engaging members of the community is key to the overall sustainability of a project. This will be discussed further in chapter five.

Key Factors in Maintaining Local Partnerships

As in any relationship, international partnerships need to be nurtured in order to continue to be fruitful. While the ultimate goal may be sustainability, a mental health training program my take many years before local entities take full ownership of the project. Indeed, the goal may be sustained partnership with the international collaborators serving in only supportive roles. Key factors in maintaining thriving international partnerships while building a mental health training program are outlined below. If one truly values collaborative partnerships, it is important to recognize and address issues of culture, expertise, power, and evaluation in your relationship with participating stakeholders.

Cultural Awareness and Sensitivity

Mental health and well-being are human rights that are often left unrealized for many in LMICs. The stigma of mental illness contributes to the high incidence of preventable or treatable disorders. An understanding of the role cultural beliefs play in how a population views mental illness is essential to creating and maintaining partnerships. When working cross-culturally, cultural humility must be employed.

Locals as Experts

While the international partners bring vast knowledge in mental health, training, consultation, and program evaluation, they are not the only experts. The local contributors must be realized for the expertise they provide. Key informants and stakeholders have the cultural and local knowledge and understanding that foreign collaborators may lack. In addition, the local partners know the local resources and the best means for accessing them.

Power Sharing

In keeping with cultural humility, and recognizing locals as experts, power sharing should be continuously practiced. The host country may lack the financial and institutional resources that the international partners possess. Nevertheless, financial power should not be used as a weapon to control the direction of the partnership or the program. In creating a mental health-training program we seek to bring about increased social and emotional wellness, with empowerment playing a key role in this.

Evaluation and Review of Goals

Maintaining partnerships involves routine evaluation and review of the goals and expectations shared by the stakeholders. The roles and responsibilities of each collaborator should be examined and commitments reaffirmed or revised as necessary. The purpose of this text is to demonstrate a model that has been successfully used in Haiti. Reviewing and evaluating goals helps answer the key questions about how successful the program is.

CONCLUSION

This chapter highlighted the key concepts related to partnership and collaboration. Using Haiti as an example, we discussed the process of engagement in an international mental health partnership. The key steps in the engagement process include: 1) Identifying community needs through data gathering, 2) meetings with stakeholders to clarify needs and expectations, and 3) developing mutual goals among partners. Taking these steps further involves immersing oneself in the culture of the host region. The local people are the most knowledgeable about the systems, values, and resources of the community. Their participation must be based on mutual respect and appreciation. The long-term success of a mental health training program requires that the local team has ownership of the program and the full capacity to carry it through. In the next chapter we will discuss the mental health training components in greater detail.

REFERENCES

Ng, C., Fraser, J., Goding, M., Paroissien, D., and Ryan, B. (2013). Partnerships for community mental health in the Aisia-Pacific: Principles and best-practice models across different sectors. *Australasian Psychiatry 21* (1), 38-45.

Ogilvie, L., Allen, M., Laryea, J., Opare, M. (2003). Building capacity through a collaborative international nursing project. *Journal of Nursing Scholarship, 35* (2), 113-118.

Sider, S. (2014). School leadership across borders: Examining a Canadian-Haitian partnership to support educational capacity-building in Haiti. *International Studies in Educational Administration 42* (1), 75-88.

Zeng, X., Hinshaw, A., Yu, M., Guo, G., and Oakley, D. (2001). Building international partnerships. *International Nursing Review, 48*, 117-121.

Chapter 5

BUILDING CAPACITY AND SUSTAINABILITY

> "What you spend years *building* may be destroyed overnight. Build anyway."
>
> *Mother Teresa*

Embarking on an international mental health capacity building project is not a matter to be undertaken lightly. It requires a strong commitment on the part of all parties involved as well as an acknowledgement that the program, which is collaboratively developed, belongs to the host country partners and should continue to be successful long after the international partnership has ended. Internationally-funded programs may end after an appointed time or abruptly—often when the international partners lose funding or change focus. An unplanned ending may lead not only to the end of the partnership, but also the end of the important work that was being done locally by the program. In this chapter, we discuss the importance of sustainability. In this chapter, we define the key factors related to sustainability and illustrate how the Mental Health Training Program in Haiti is working towards maintaining long-term sustainable programing.

The question of sustainability is not unique to international mental health partnerships. The public health and medical communities have a long history of engaging in international projects in Low- and Middle-income Countries (LMICs; George & Meadows-Oliver, 2013). As such, the question of sustainability naturally arises. In their review of literature related to international nursing partnerships, George and Meadows-Oliver noted that of the nine articles reviewed, four articles discussed phasing out the participation of high-income countries (HIC) as part of a sustainability plan. Two of those studies focused on the use of a train-the-trainer model towards meeting this goal.

In a critical review of literature related to sustainability, Hudson and Vissing (2013) found that the "the concept has been overgeneralized and has become a buzzword" in the healthcare arenas (p.1). The varying definitions often are linked to a particular agenda, not necessarily focusing on what exactly is to be sustained and how it is to be assessed and evaluated over time. As one develops programs in LMICs, it is vital to jointly define sustainability and outline the step by step objectives necessary in achieving this goal.

The models and frameworks established in the medical field have many key points transferable towards building sustainability in international mental health capacity building programs. The Conceptual Model for Partnership and Sustainability in Global Health Framework, provided by Leffers and Mitchell (2011), recognizes many similar factors as those discussed in this monograph. The model was developed as a result of grounded theory research with nurses from the United States who participated in international health programs. Emergent themes related to sustainability included "partnership, leadership, ownership, quality of collaboration, capacity building, and resource availability" (Leffers & Mitchell, 2011, p. 94). Like many others, the authors recognize that sustainability of any program resulting from an international partnership must include local empowerment and capacity building.

In this monograph, we argue that sustainability is the ability for a program to continue at a local level without the sole reliance on international partners' knowledge or expertise, physical presence, and financing. This does not imply that international partners may not continue to engage on some level. It does, however, mean that the local stakeholders are empowered in making decisions, planning, delivering, and evaluating their program according to the changing needs of those being served. The international partners, as well as local partners, may change and grow. Resources may be lost, but new strategies need to be developed to keep the program active. Sustainability or longevity relies on three key resources: financial, knowledge, and human capital. By building capacity at the local and systemic levels, the long-term sustainability of the program can be achieved.

Financial resources are often seen as the major requirement in creating and sustaining programs (George & Meadows-Oliver, 2013). Many international programs in LMICs rely on the financial resources from the partner country. This may be in the form of donations, grants, and/or fundraising. U.S.-based partners may volunteer their time and service to the program, even paying for their own travel and accommodations during their time in the host country. Even in the absence of visits from international partners, financial resources are needed to run the program. Funds for securing training sites, catering for food services, and providing transportation are only some of the possible expenses. Depending on the structure of the program, stipends or salaries may also be necessary. A mental health training program, as with other types of programs, will also require concrete materials in order to fulfill the program needs. Brochures, manuals, and other educational materials will need to be provided for trainers and participants.

A mental health program involves extensive knowledge resources. Initially, the internationally-based partners may take the lead in providing the knowledge of mental health. While it may be challenging to identify mental health professionals and facilities in LMICs, the structure for sustaining ongoing knowledge building and overall capacity building must be included when creating the program (e.g., via a "train-the-trainer" model). Furthermore, the cultural knowledge and local expertise of the in-country partners should be honored and leveraged. The Mental Health Training Program in Haiti involved mental health professionals from the United States who trained local people to be trainers of the curriculum. The in-country trainers continue to address cultural elements and emerging needs of the community by evaluating and revising the curriculum. This may be done in partnership with mental health experts, but it is initiated by the local training teams.

We argue that human capital is the most valuable resource for sustaining a mental health training program. As discussed throughout this monograph, the local partners are essential to the success of any program. Using a capacity-building model shares the knowledge resources of international partners and creates a sustainable training team of local people. Hence, international partners move from being essential to serving in an advisory or complementary capacity. Furthermore, in building partnerships locally, the training teams will be able to accesses reliable networks of people to accomplish their goals.

LESSONS FROM HAITI

Local sustainability is the ultimate goal of the Mental Health Training Program in Haiti. The international partners were initially involved through a process of meeting with key informants and stakeholders. Intensive and purposeful planning helped establish concrete goals and objectives for addressing the growing need for mental health training in Haiti. The Mental Health Training Program was enacted as an intervention in the Cap-Haitien and Arcahaie regions. The international training team invested hundreds of hours in developing the program in these sites. Now, the power of the program lies in the hands of the local people.

SUSTAINABILITY AND BUILDING LOCAL CAPACITY

Chapter two provided details of the Mental Health Training Program. In both regions, the train-the-trainer model was used. This model ensures that knowledge resources and human resources can be sustained locally. In our implementation of the train-the-trainer model, the partnership principles of power-sharing and valuing locals as experts are actualized through transparent processes and coaching. Trainers are linked with local partners in order to access resources such as training sites, food services, and program materials. The curriculum has been continuously updated to reflect the local dialects and nuances. The local partners provide the resource of cultural knowledge for doing this. Again, as a principle of partnership, the program is continuously evaluated and culturally enhanced.

The purpose of using this training model is to create a team of individuals who can facilitate the continuation of the program without extensive external resources. Efforts in building the program have concentrated on building local partnerships. As discussed earlier, the local resources are often richer than international partners might assume. Engaging key stakeholders and seeking non-traditional partnerships have been essential to the success of the Mental Health Training Program in Haiti.

The program has focused on developing and enhancing leadership capacity among the training teams. The trainers are carefully selected for their knowledge of the training material, demonstration of leadership, and willingness to serve the community. The training teams are made up solely of volunteers. The partnerships with the hospital and schools assures that individual trainers will have the time away from work to train others and engage in community service to promote mental health knowledge and well-being.

In Cap-Haitien, the trainers have named themselves *The Mental Health Training Team of the North*. In Arcahaie, it is *Team Unity* that leads the trainings in this region of the country. The training teams take ownership of the program in the following ways:

1. Teach the Mental Health Training Program Curriculum to new participants in their respective communities.
2. Conduct local workshops on mental health and well-being in the larger community.
3. Host radio programming to provide community education on mental health and social well-being.
4. Create public service announcements to be used in the local media.
5. Conduct presentations at local schools, churches, and organizations to further create social awareness of mental health issues and lessen social stigma within the community.
6. Train new trainers who are selected from participants in the trainings provided.
7. Act as a self-governing body with regular planning meetings.
8. Maintain systems of communication between local trainers and international partners serving as consultants.
9. Plan, organize, and implement all training sessions.
10. Manage all logistics of the training sessions, including ordering training materials; arranging sites, transportation, and catering; and recruiting program participants.

The individual trainers also leverage their own networks and resources. In Arcahaie, for example, members who are school leaders offer space in their schools or local community centers as training sites. They access nearby restaurants and engage them as partners who can provide discounts or donations for training lunches. They engage grantors within the country to fund the cost of printing training materials. The teams have been successful in implementing the training program using the financial, knowledge, and human resources available at the local level. Ultimately, the power of this model has been the selection and training of a committed and talented group of volunteers.

SUSTAINABILITY AND BUILDING CAPACITY SYSTEMICALLY

The Mental Health Training Program in Haiti began with a small team of U.S.-based trainers led by the first author, Guerda Nicolas. In order to ensure that the training teams would continue to have the resources that international partnership can provide, the program was linked to an organization made up of Haitian mental health and development professionals from Haiti, the United States, and Canada. Rebâti Santé Mentale (RSM) is a non-profit organization committed to building mental health systems in Haiti.

RSM members initially toured the regions and met with local partners, engaging in the process of partnership and community building. RSM identified its contribution as serving as a financial resource to local leaders. RSM members continue to use their expertise to conduct fundraising and participate in grant seeking to help fund the Mental Health Training Program. RSM also contributes knowledge resources in the form of training to trainers to further build their mental health knowledge and leadership capacity. The human resources of training staff and consultants are also provided regularly to the trainers. RSM also maintains relationships with the local stakeholders and partners.

Rebâti Santé Mentale builds partnerships with other organizations and groups, which can then be leveraged for the training teams. For example, a partnership with the Haitian Mental Health Network (HMHN) has contributed to HMHN members serving as trainers and consultants to the training teams. RSM's various University partners have provided the support of students to assist on projects and fundraising activities for the Program. RSM also engages in other Haiti-based mental health initiatives, demonstrating an investment to this project in the long-term.

CONCLUSION

Sustainability should be the ultimate goal of an international mental health partnership. Programs that solely rely on the expertise and human capital of foreign partners working in LMIC sites may end when the partners lose funding or find other projects that attract them. This can leave the local programs without the financial, knowledge, or human resources to continue to provide services to the local community. Guided by the key principle of community partnership, the train-the-trainer model used in the Mental Health Training Program in Haiti builds the local capacity for sustaining the program. Furthermore, the engagement of an organization whose charge is to provide resources for sustainability is important. Besides engaging in fundraising and providing consultants and trainers, there is a sharing of knowledge so that team leaders can also build valuable skills towards local sustainability.

REFERENCES

George, E., & Meadows-Oliver, M. (2013). Searching for collaboration in international nursing partnerships: A literature review. *International Nursing Review, 60*(1), 31-36.

Hudson, C., & Vissing, Y. (2013). Sustainability at the edge of chaos: Its limits and possibilities in public health. *Biomed Research International.* http://dx.doi.org/10.1155/2013/801614.

Leffers, J., & Mitchell, E. (2010). Conceptual model for partnership and sustainability in global health. *Public Health Nursing. 28*(1), 91–102.

Chapter 6

EVALUATION OF THE MENTAL HEALTH PROGRAM IN HAITI

> "We mean well, our motives are good, but we have neglected to conduct care-full due diligence to determine emotional, economic, and cultural outcomes on the receiving end of our charity. Why do we miss this crucial aspect in evaluating our charitable work? Because, as compassionate people, we have been evaluating our charity by the rewards we receive through service, rather than the benefits received by the served."
>
> *Robert Lupton, Toxic Charity*

> "Everything that can be counted does not necessarily count; everything that counts cannot necessarily be counted"
>
> *Albert Einstein*

Although there are reportedly many mental health training programs occurring worldwide—and particularly in low- and middle-income countries (LMICs)—few of these programs include a systematic evaluation plan. Nevertheless, it is without argument that a sound evaluation program should be the cornerstone of all programs, especially international ones. Evaluation, loosely described as systematic investigation of whether a program is working or not, has changed over the years in terms of methodology and approach. More broadly, evaluation is often defined as "the systematic application of scientific methods to assess the design, implementation, improvement or outcomes of a program" (Rossi & Freeman, 1993).

Developing programs without an integrated evaluation plan embedded into the program does not facilitate the creation of a sustainable program. Recognizing the importance of creating a training program in Haiti that would be long lasting, evaluating the impact of the project and detailing lessons learned in implementation of the program were of high priority during the planning stages. Doing so would enable us to both feed the information back into the program (and thus improve its quality) as a well as disseminate it to other LMICs that might benefit from similar programs and processes. Elements incorporated into evaluation of the Haiti Mental Health Training Program (HMHTP) include:

1. Administration of pre- and post-test questionnaires to collect data on mental health knowledge of and psychological distress
2. Assessment of competencies gained through training
3. Measures of participants' satisfaction with training and services.

Through the integration of such an evaluation, we have learned valuable information that has led to the improvement of the Mental Health Training Program in Haiti. In this chapter, we provide an overview of the approaches and methods used in conducting an evaluation of a program, highlights from the process used in the HMHTP, and lessons learned over the years.

OVERVIEW OF PROGRAM EVALUATION

Program evaluation provides an opportunity to demonstrate what is working helps to improve the overall quality of the program. There is an extensive body of research on different methods and approaches that one can use to conduct an effective evaluation of one's project (Donaldson, Christie, & Mark, 2009; Nutbeam & Bauman, 2011). There are many benefits of undertaking such a process, the main one being that evaluation of programs or projects provides an opportunity for understanding and improvement of the project using strategies shown to be useful, doable, relevant, and accurate. Thus, one must be mindful of selecting the type of evaluation that fits the project in order to ensure the method is appropriate for the specific project being implemented.

TYPES OF EVALUATION

There are several types of evaluation approaches that one can choose from in evaluating a program, including:

Context evaluation: Investigating how the program can or does operate in particular environments in terms of social, political, physical, and economic factors. This type of evaluation could include a community needs or organizational assessment and may include sample questions such as, "What are the environmental barriers to accessing program services?" (W.K. Kellogg Foundation, 2004).

Formative evaluation: Assessing the needs that a new program should fulfill (Short, Hennessy, & Campbell, 1996), examining the early stages of a program's development (Rossi & Freeman, 1993), or testing a program on a small scale before broad dissemination (Coyle, Boruch, & Turner, 1991). A sample question of this type of evaluation is, "Who is the intended audience for the program?"

Process evaluation: Examining the implementation and operation of program components. This is key to understanding the various aspects of program outcomes, both successful and unsuccessful. A sample question might be, "Was the program administered as planned?"

Impact evaluation: This type of evaluation is used to examine the magnitude of both positive and negative changes produced by a program (Rossi & Freeman, 1993). This may include both immediately upon the implementation of the program or throughout the program (Green & Kreuter, 1991), an example question that this type o evaluation might seek to answer is, "Did the participant's knowledge change after attending the program?" This is the type of evaluation used in the Mental Health Training program in Haiti described below.

Outcome evaluation: Assessing the short and long-term results of a program. Sample question: What are the short-term and long-term positive effects of program participation?

Performance or program monitoring: Similar to process evaluation, but differs in that it provides regular updates of evaluation results to stakeholders rather than summarizing results at the evaluation's conclusion (Burt, Harrell, Newmark, Aron, & Jacobs, 1997; Rossi & Freeman, 1993).

EVALUATION STANDARDS AND DESIGNS

Evaluation should be incorporated during the initial stages of program development. Initially, being able to describe the program in detail is key. Making this a collaborative activity can create a mutual understanding of the program, the evaluation process, and various terminology and techniques. Developing a program description also helps ensure that program activities and objectives are clearly defined and measurable. Evaluation should be five things: feasible, useful, culturally competent, ethical, and accurate (Centers for Disease Control and Prevention, 1999). Data should be collected over time using multiple instruments that are valid (measuring what they are intended to) and reliable (consistently producing similar results; Rossi & Freeman, 1993). The use of qualitative as well as quantitative data can also provide a more comprehensive picture of the program.

Steps in Conducting an Evaluation

The program evaluation process can be a complex and complicated aspect of the implementation of any project. As such, the planning phase is one of the most important steps in ensuring that your program evaluation is effective. This stage is likely to guide all other aspects of the project. Throughout the literature, there are many models with a varying number of steps. The literature on the different approaches and methods can be daunting. Nevertheless, the process can be guided by the following key questions:

What are you planning to evaluate? This process involves creating a separate and dedicated document for the evaluation of the project. This document should have the following key items included: title and description of the program, selection criteria for eligibility, and factors outside of the project that might impact the program.

What is the purpose of the proposed evaluation? It is very important to clearly state the main purposes of the evaluation plan for the project. Doing so ensures that all who are involved in the process get a chance to communicate their needs and understanding. More importantly, this step enables you to arrive at some key questions that are driving the evaluation process and the type of evaluation (formative or summative) that is best to answer these questions.

Who will use the evaluation? Part of the evaluation process is determining who will access the evaluation and who will use the information obtained from it. Understanding the target audience will ensure that the materials are presented in ways that are easily digested.

How will they use it? Not only is it important for the analysis to be completed by an organization with a reputable research background and from a neutral standpoint, it is also imperative that it addresses all the questions that key stakeholders may have. After identifying audiences and stakeholders, an important step is to work collaboratively to shape the questions being asked, determine the way(s) in which the results will be communicated, and decide what the tone, applicability, and actionable advice of the results should look like.

What key research question(s) will the evaluation seek to answer? Once the purpose is clearly articulated, a set of questions can be created that will serve as the guide for the scope of the project and enable the team to prioritize the analysis and recommendations in the final report.

When is the evaluation needed? Moving forward with the evaluation plan, it is critical to have a realistic timeline indicating what will be done by when and by whom.

Who will be responsible for each stage? When will each stage be completed? Given the complexity of the evaluation process, it is very important to clearly lay out who is leading which aspects of the process early on. This will enable you to identify any breakdowns in the process and make any corrections necessary to complete the evaluation on a timely manner.

Use of Logic Models

Most program evaluation begins with the creation of a logic model that can serve to clarify program elements and expectations for the stakeholders. By clearly outlining the steps, inputs, activities and outputs in a diagram, the logic model can make sure that the right data is collected to answer the specific questions sought to answer through the project (CDC, 1999).

Communicating Evaluation Findings

It is important to be mindful of the audience that will be recipient of the final evaluation report. The report should be disseminated to the director of the project and the team members associated with the project. In addition to these individuals, the findings might be shared with important stakeholders associated with the project. As such, an executive summary of the report that is clear, brief, and to the point should be created and disseminated to these individuals. Ultimately, it is important to create a report that is tailored to the audience.

Evaluation Approach for Haiti Mental Training Program

The Haiti Mental Health Training Program, described in more detail in Chapter 4, has been implemented in two different geographical regions of the country: Cap Haitien and Arcahaie. In this section, a description of the evaluation process used in both locales is provided, with Cap Haitien as the main illustrating example.

Setting and Participants

Setting in Cap Haitien. Cap Haitien is Haiti's second largest city (population approximately 200,000) and has the nation's second largest health center, the *Hôpital Universitaire Justinien* (HUJ). The HUJ is the sole hospital serving Cap Haitien and is also the referral hospital for the entire Northern Health Department of Haiti, serving a population of 1 million people. The HUJ is an academic center affiliated with three medical schools in Haiti and a school of nursing which is located adjacent to the hospital. HUJ has the full range of medical services including family medicine, internal medicine, pediatrics, orthopedics, obstetrics and gynecology, general surgery, anesthesiology, orthopedics, otolaryngology and ophthalmology and a preventive/Public Health unit. The HUJ has 35 physicians and 100 nurses.

Cap Haitien Participants. In Cap Haitien, 113 local health providers (nurses, physicians, social workers, and others) were trained to identify, triage, and provide supportive services for mental health disorders. These professionals included those located in the urban area of Cap Haitien as well as rural areas in the vicinity. The trainings were conducted in four cohorts of 25-30 trainees who met for five days for a total of forty hours of training during a one-week period. Two additional trainees began the program but did not complete. The remaining 113 trainees had full retention in the program and participated in all aspects.

Of the 113 trainees, 13 participated in the "train the trainer" program. These trainers received additional didactic and workshop sessions on the program content as well as on pedagogical matters. Each trainer had two levels of hands-on experience in administering the 5-day training program–one time as junior facilitators and the second time as senior facilitators—both times under supervision of University of Miami program staff.

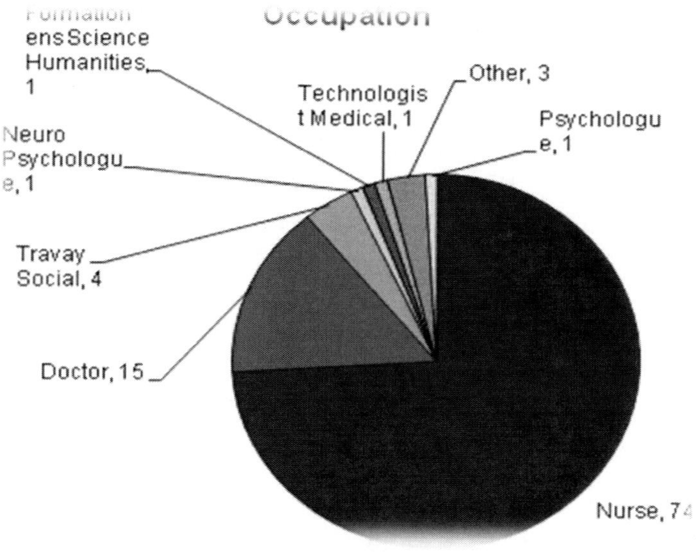

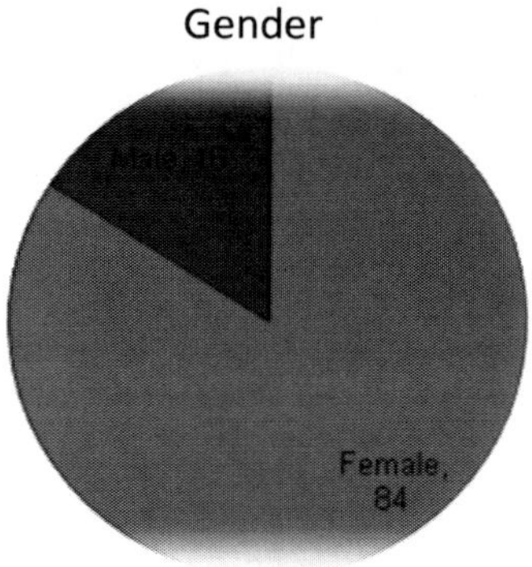

Evaluation Process and Materials

The impact evaluation of the HMHTP included quantitative and qualitative measures of impact and satisfaction from trainees, as well as from local trainers, health care supervisors, and administrators. In addition to these assessment documents, we conducted observations of the participants throughout the week of the training program via their small group presentations, questions, and periodic concerns brought up about aspects of the program.

Quantitative Assessment

The training program has a built-in evaluation component used to gauge trainee progress. Personnel are evaluated on their knowledge base and awareness of psychological issues at the beginning of the training, midway through program, and at program completion, using quantifiable questionnaires. The questionnaires were developed for Haitian participants in Haiti. At the beginning of the program, each participant is asked to complete the following questionnaires:

1. *Questions* - This is an open ended questionnaire created to ask participants questions regarding their perceptions about mental health, mental illnesses, grief, etc. This questionnaire allowed us to gauge the participants' initial beliefs about the various topics discussed throughout the training.
2. *Demographic Questions* - This is a likert-type scale that asks common demographic information about the participants in terms of age, marital and employment status, language use, years in their profession, etc. The information obtained on this form enabled us to determine if any of the measured results differed across demographic variables. For example, did belief about mental health differ across marital status?
3. *Pre-assessment Knowledge Questionnaire* - This measure was created to ensure that the presentations were geared appropriately to the individuals attending the training, as well as to test participants' knowledge base prior to and after the training session. The questionnaire consisted of a list of content areas; participants were instructed to check off the ones with which they were already familiar.

On the last day of the training, the participants are given an open-ended short answer examination that focused on the content covered during the week. In addition to the exam, each group was asked to present on a subject that they selected during the week and prepared as a team. Each member of the team was required to have a speaking role and members were evaluated using a presentation rating rubric developed for the purpose of the project (see appendix A). The documents are used throughout the week to determine and select individuals whom the team felt might be excellent candidates as trainers in the program. Lastly, each participant is asked to complete a program evaluation form that consisted of questions pertaining to knowledge gained, content and structure of the program, and overall satisfaction with the training program.

Focus Groups

Focus groups were conducted at the end of the project to evaluate program acceptability and to gain recommendations for future work—one group with eight trainees and one with eight trainers. In addition, key informant interviews were conducted with two administrators and clinical leaders. Preliminary findings of the qualitative evaluation components indicate that the program was very well accepted at all levels—from trainees to local health leaders—and that there is a desire and perceived need to expand the program to other areas of Haiti. There was significant buy-in from local authorities who had referred trainees to the program and gave them paid release time to attend project activities. The following quotes were translated from French to English from the evaluation forms of the participants.

> "I thank all the trainers for this great training session in Mental Health..."
>
> "We would like to continue with the training."
>
> "The team was very competent and I would like to participate in another Health training very soon."
>
> "The program is really informative. I congratulate the trainers of various teams Miami and Haiti. A thousand thank you and congratulations!"
>
> "This was a rather rich experience, but sadly was too short."
>
> "I like the way the training was given. It was very useful for us and the other members of the society such as the health personnel."

Trainer Observations of Participants

In addition to quantitative and qualitative approaches, the five days of training provided ample opportunities to observe the participants—through their work in small group activities, presentations to the whole group, and overall behavior in the group. This process is conducted by the trainers throughout the week of the training and served as additional data for the selection of potential trainers.

Conclusion

Including an evaluation of the Haiti Mental Health Training Program has been and continues to be a very important aspect of the project. The evaluation process enables us to understand the overall impact of the program on the participants and determine if the program was effective. This is even more important as we are training local trainers who can continue to implement the program in their respective communities. Indeed, the information gained through the process enables us to make changes to the program, which has made the program stronger and culturally relevant.

Of note, there are some things that the evaluation approached used could not capture—one such aspect is personal growth. Although we set out to evaluate impact of the program with respect to the knowledge gain pre- and post-training, we did not anticipated the high rate of personal growth reported by participants across both sites. Through the informational interviews with participants, we learned of the many ways that participating in the program enriched their intra and interpersonal relationships. Specifically, the participants highlighted a greater awareness of their own emotions, reactions to events and people in their lives, and their ability to manage stress better. Interpersonally, the participants discussed improvements in their relationships with their partners and their children as a result of their participant in the training program. Further qualitative and quantitative analyses are ongoing and manuscripts for publication are in preparation.

References

Burt, M. R., Harrell, A. V., Newmark, L. C., Aron, L. Y., & Jacobs, L. K. (1997). *Evaluation guidebook: Projects funded by S.T.O.P. formula grants under the Violence Against Women Act.* Washington, DC: The Urban Institute.

Centers for Disease Control and Prevention. (1999). Framework for program evaluation in public health. *MMWR Recommendations and Reports, 48*(RR11), 1-40.

Chalk, R., & King, P. A. (Eds.). (1998). *Violence in families: Assessing prevention and treatment programs.* Washington DC: National Academy Press.

Coyle, S. L., Boruch, R. F., & Turner, C. F. (Eds.). (1991). *Evaluating AIDS prevention programs: Expanded edition*. Washington DC: National Academy Press.

Donaldson, S., Christie, C., Mark, M. (eds), 2009, What counts as credible evidence in applied research and evaluation practice?, Sage Publications, California.

Green, L.W., & Kreuter, M. W. (1991). *Health promotion planning: An educational and environmental approach* (2nd ed.). Mountain View, CA: Mayfield Publishing Company.

National Committee for Injury Prevention and Control. (1989). Injury prevention: Meeting the challenge. *American Journal of Preventive Medicine, 5*(Suppl. 3).

Nutbeam, D., Bauman, A., 2011, Evaluation in a nutshell: a practical guide to the evaluation of health promotion programs, McGraw Hill, North Ryde.

Rossi, P. H., & Freeman, H. E. (1993). *Evaluation: A systematic approach* (5th ed.). Newbury Park, CA: Sage Publications, Inc.

Short, L., Hennessy, M., & Campbell, J. (1996). Tracking the work. In M. Witmer (Ed.), *Family violence: Building a coordinated community response: A guide for communities*. Washington, DC: American Medical Association.

W.K. Kellogg Foundation. (2004). W.K. Kellogg evaluation handbook. Retrieved from: https://www.wkkf.org/resource-directory/resource/2010/w-k-kellogg-foundation-evaluation-handbook.

Chapter 7

CONCLUSION: IMPLICATIONS FOR GLOBAL MENTAL HEALTH TRAINING PROGRAMS

"In the long history of humankind (and animal kind, too) those who learned to collaborate and improvise most effectively have prevailed."
Charles Darwin

At a recent international conference, the question was posed as to whether mental health workers can work "without borders," similar to what some of our colleagues in medicine are doing (i.e., *Doctors Without Borders*). After extensive discussion, the participants concluded that the elements (trust, alliance, culture, etc.) of the work required by a mental health worker do not lend themselves to effectively working without borders. Having said that, it is recognized that over the last several years, we have witnessed an increasing number of disasters across the globe. Such events are even more devastating for countries with limited resources. Thus, the need for humanitarian efforts are even greater for many of these countries. Although it is noble to leave one's space of comfort to travel remotely to provide assistance to those in need, a "without borders" approach to mental health intervention may not be the best strategy. Given the importance of trust and relationship in the work that mental health professionals do, it is necessary for us to pause before flying to another country to provide service. Working internationally requires careful planning and execution in order for them to be efficient and effective.

Using our experiences over the last two decades working collaboratively to develop and implement a mental health training program in Haiti, we wanted to create this monograph as a resource for those who are embarking on and thinking about that work. We are by no means the only group who is engaging in this work and many others such as Heppner and colleagues (Heppner, Warmpold, Owen, Mindi, & Wang, 2015), are doing similar work and suggest that one does as much reading as necessary prior to engaging in this work. Through this monograph, we sought to provide an overview of five key areas using Haiti as an opportunity to illustrate each of the points. The ideas that we discussed in this monograph have been studied by other researchers and these studies served as a good foundation and validation of the work that we are doing in Haiti. An overview of the literature for each of the elements is provided to guide your own decision making as you move forward. Below is a summary of the key areas that we discussed in this book.

THE MENTAL HEALTH TRAINING PROGRAM

This book opened with an overview of the mental health training program that we have developed and implemented in Haiti over the years. Through this chapter, we sought to demonstrate the ways that the curriculum was developed to reflect the culture in which we worked as well as to integrate the capacity-building initiative in the training from the outset. The creation of the training manual and trainers manual was grounded in a community empowerment framework and thus seeks to ensure that the community is actively engaged in the development and implementation of the program. Ultimately, we want the communities in which we work to become the owner of the project while we serve as consultants to the local teams.

THE GUIDING PRINCIPLES

As we embarked in this work a little over two decades ago, we wanted to make sure that we had a good framework that would serve as a foundation for the work that we are doing. The field of community psychology—with its focus on strength and well-being versus pathology, and community building and capacity building as opposed to individual building—served as the foundation from which to build our work. The principles described in Chapter 3 are a reflection of the work many community psychologists do, integrated with our own cultural understanding and knowledge of Haiti. We found these principles to be particularly useful in a collectivistic society such as Haiti, where the needs of the collective supersede the individual needs. The seven core principles that guided the development and implementation of the mental health-training program are:

(1) Developing In-Country Partnerships
(2) Enhancing Cultural Knowledge
(3) Conducting a Community Needs Assessment
(4) Selecting a Culturally Relevant Team
(5) Creating a Culturally Relevant Curriculum
(6) Conducting a Program Evaluation
(7) Building Local Capacity.

In this monograph, we provided an overview of each of the seven principles and highlighted field examples from Haiti that we hope have illustrated each of these principles. Given the importance of principle 1 (building local partnership) and 2 (building local capacity), we have dedicated specific chapters to these principles in order to provide more detailed information and examples of each.

BUILDING LOCAL PARTNERSHIP

As we have indicated throughout the book, the bedrock of the training program in Haiti centers on the partnerships formed with the local communities in which the program has been implemented. We cannot stress this point enough. In order to ensure that the program is integrated within the community, the local partners must be involved from conceptualization, to implementation, and through evaluation. Through such a process, the members of the community are more likely to see the program as their own and, thus, as something to which they are willing to dedicate time and resources in order to ensure its success.

In Chapter 4 of this monograph, we provided an overview regarding the process of building partnership for a program and highlighted some of the ways that we built those partnerships in the communities in which the program is run. Building and promoting true partnership involves engaging these partners earlier on in the process and empowering the community. What is noteworthy is that while the framework is the same, the process and the partners involved from one community to the next differs. Thus, there is no "one size fits all" approach when it comes to building partnership locally. The partnerships might be unconventional, such as being open to partnering with numerous different groups. Extensive understanding of the communities of interest is needed in order to determine the specific community partners that are central to the development and execution of the program. In order words, building a self-sufficient local team is central to operating a successful program internationally.

BUILDING CAPACITY

One of the key questions that we often asked ourselves as we embarked on a new program cycle or in new community is what happens to the project if something happens to us? If the answer to this question is that the project goes with us, then we know that we are off track and need to reevaluate the program. Ultimately, we seek to create programs that are embedded in the community and build on the strengths and skills of the people within the community. Thus, we see the work as building on the existing strengths of the people and community and ensuring that the program is able to continue beyond our time. This is how we envision the concept of sustainability being actualized. As such, embedded in the program is the integration of the train-the-trainer model that allows us to select individuals with the skills and conviction to move the program forward. From the first training session of the program we are building a team of trainers that will be capable of continuing the program with limited assistance from us as the project moves forward. As a result, there is a team of trainers in each of the areas in which we have worked who are continuing the program through workshops, presentations, radio appearances, etc. More importantly, as the program progresses, we want this team of trainers to be the public face of the Mental Health Training Program—not us.

In addition to building capacity locally, we felt that it was important to ensure that we also build the *international* capacity that can serve as the link between the various teams of the project. *Rebati Sante Mentale* was created as an organization that can be long standing and serve as the connector for these teams. Although the overall vision and mission of *Rebati Sante Mentale* is to work in partnership with the Haitian Ministry of Health to establish and implement an effective mental health plan throughout the country, its link to the various community teams legitimizes the organization and the work of the team members.

EVALUATION

In this monograph we provided an overview of the evaluation methods and process that we used to evaluate the mental health training program in Haiti. The research on program evaluation highlights the importance of ensuring that the following four key elements are addressed: utility, feasibility, propriety, and accuracy (Fitzpatrick, Sanders, & Worthen, 2011; Yarbrough, Shulha, Hopson, and Caruthers, 2011). In sum, the literature indicates that the evaluation must be useful to the stakeholders, doable, reflective of and owned by the local community, and reflective of the program in question.

Following the appropriate steps of program evaluation, we wanted to make sure that we created an evaluation method that can be easily replicated and understood by the local teams. Therefore, we ensured that the forms and questionnaires that we used were reflective of the local community and were clearly understood by the trainers of the program. In doing so, we engaged the trainers in the evaluation process throughout the training meetings to ensure that they know what types of measures to implement at what points during the training. More importantly, we want to be confident that the trainers know what to do once the data are collected and how best to utilize the data to further improve the program. Ultimately, we have seen the importance of collecting data not to meet a grant requirement or other demands, but to create an evaluation plan and process that is going to be useful to the program, trainers, and the stakeholders.

We by no means believe that our approach is the "right" or only model; we are simply sharing what we have learned through our work in Haiti for over 20 years. We hope that this information is useful to other mental health professionals seeking to do similar work. It is our hope that the information provided in this monograph will serve as a guide and example to many who are looking to create similar collaborative partnerships in different countries.

REFERENCES

Fitzpatrick, J. L., Sanders, J. R., & Worthen, B. R. (2011). *Program evaluation: Alternative approaches and practical guidelines* (4th Ed.). Upper Saddle River, NJ: Pearson Education, Inc.

Hepner, P. P., Warmpold, B. E., Owen, J., Mindi, T. N., & Wang, K. T. (2015). *Research design in counseling* (4th Ed.). Boston, MA: Cengage Learning, Inc.

Yarbrough, D. B., Shulha, L. M., Hopson, R. K., & Caruthers, F. A. (2011). *The program evaluation standards: A guide for evaluators and evaluation users* (3rd ed.). Thousand Oaks, CA: Sage.

About the Authors

Dr. *Guerda Nicolas*, is a licensed clinical psychologist and Assistant Director of the Institute for the Study and Promotion of Race and Culture (ISPRC) along with Dr. Janet E. Helms. She is also a Professor at the University of Miami in the School of Education and Human Development, in the Department of Educational Psychological Studies. She obtained her doctoral degree in clinical psychology from Boston University. She completed her predoctoral training at Columbia University Medical Center and her postdoctoral training the New York State Psychiatric Institute/Columbia University, Department of Child Psychiatry. As a multicultural (Haitian American) and multilingual psychologist (Spanish, French, and Haitian Creole), her research is reflective of her background and interests. Her current research projects focus on developing spirituality across the life span among ethnic minorities, culturally effective mental health intervention for ethnic minority adolescents, with a specific focus on Immigrant children, adolescents, and families. In addition, she conducts research on social support networks of Caribbean with a specific focus on Haitians. She has published several articles and book chapters and delivered numerous invited presentations at the national and international conferences in the areas of women issues, depression and intervention among Haitians, social support networks of ethnic minorities, and spirituality. Her recent books include, Social Networks and the Mental Health of Haitian Immigrants (2011) and Contemporary Parenting Practices: A Global Perspective (2015).

nguerda@miami.edu

Dr. *Gemima St. Louis* is an Associate Professor in the Clinical Psychology Department at William James College (WJC). She is the Co-Director of the

Center for Multicultural & Global Mental Health, the Director of the African & Caribbean Mental Health Concentration, and a Faculty Member in the Concentration on Children and Families of Adversity and Resilience at WJC. She is also the Director of the *PATHWAYS Program*, a school-based initiative that provides trauma-focused, evidence-informed mental health services to urban youth in the Boston Public Schools. Her primary clinical and research focus is on ethnically-diverse children, adolescents, and families with histories of trauma, chronic diseases, and behavioral and emotional challenges. Dr. St. Louis has developed culturally-sensitive psychoeducational programs for youth and women, and has conducted research on trauma and HIV disease among ethnic minority and immigrant groups. Dr. St. Louis is the Past-President of the Boston-based Haitian Mental Health Network and an alumna of the American Psychological Association's Leadership Institute for Women in Psychology. She is actively engaged in leading service learning and mental health capacity-building programs in Haiti.

Dr. *Castagna Lacet* is an Assistant Professor in the School of Social Work at Bridgewater State University in Massachusetts. She received her masters and doctorate in social work at Boston College in the Graduate School of Social Work. Dr. Lacet's social work practice and consultation has focused on at-risk youth, families affected by family violence, and the mental health needs of the Haitian community. She serves as the President of the Haitian Mental Health Network, a collaborative of mental health providers working locally and in Haiti to build mental health capacity, and to raise awareness and decrease stigma about mental illness in the Haitian community. Dr. Lacet's teaching includes courses in research methods, social work practice, and human diversity. Her research areas focus on the mental health and well-being of Haitians, capacity building, and developing cross-cultural allyship within the social work profession.

INDEX

D

E

F

S

T

U

V

W